Acta Hæmatologica

Founded 1948 by E. Meulengracht, K. Rohr, and G. Rosenow
Continued by H. Lüdin (1960–1977), U. Bucher (1977–1983), R.S. Hillman (1978–1987), H.R. Marti (1983–1988), E.A. Beck (1984–1988)

General Information

Publication data: 'Acta Haematologica' is published 8 times annually. Volumes 85–86 with 4 issues each appear in 1991.

Subscription rates: Subscriptions run for a full calendar year. Prices are given per volume, surface postage included.

Personal subscription: SFr. 238.–, US$ 190.40. (Must be in the name of, billed to, and paid by an individual. Order must be marked 'personal subscription'.)

Institutional subscription: SFr. 340.–, US$ 272.00. (Regular rate.)

Members of the Int. Soc. of Haematology SFr. 204.–, US$ 163.20.

Airmail postage: SFr. 25.–, US$ 18.00. (Extra per volume.)

Microform subscription: SFr. 170.–, US$ 136.00. (Available exclusively to subscribers of the paper edition.)

Single issues and back volumes: Information on availability and prices can be obtained through the Publisher.

Subscription orders: Orders can be placed at agencies, bookstores, directly with the Publisher S. Karger AG, P.O. Box, CH – 4009 Basel (Switzerland) or with any of the following distributors:

Deutschland, Österreich, Ost-Europa:
S. Karger GmbH, Postfach 1724
D-W – 8034 Germering/München

France: Librairie Luginbühl
36, bd de Latour-Maubourg, F – 75007 Paris

Great Britain, Ireland:
S. Karger Publishers, 11 Ravenscroft Road
Beckenham, Kent BR3 4TP

USA: S. Karger Publishers, Inc.
26 West Avon Road, P.O. Box 529
Farmington, CT 06085

India, Bangladesh, Sri Lanka:
S. Karger India Subscription Agency
B – 5/132 Safdarjung Enclave
New Delhi-110029

Japan: Katakura Libri, Inc.
36-9 Hongo 3-chome, Bunkyo-ku, Tokyo 113

Change of address: Both old and new address should be stated and sent to the subscription source.

KARGER

Bibliographic indices: This journal is regularly listed in bibliographic services, including *Current Contents®*.

Book Reviews: Books are accepted for review by special agreement.

Advertising: Correspondence and rate requests should be addressed to the Publisher.

Acta Haematol
Printed in Switzerland

S. Karger AG,
Postfach, CH – 4009 Basel (Schweiz)

Erscheint anderthalbmonatlich;
pro Jahr 2 Bände zu 4 Heften

Submission: Only original papers written in English are considered and should be sent to:
Prof. Dr. B. Ramot
S. Karger AG
Editorial Office 'Acta Haematologica'
P.O. Box
CH – 4009 Basel (Switzerland)
Manuscripts should be submitted in triplicate (with three sets of illustrations of which one is an original), typewritten double-spaced on one side of the paper, with a wide margin.

Conditions: All manuscripts are subject to editorial review. Manuscripts are received with the explicit understanding that they are not under simultaneous consideration by any other publication. Submission of an article for publication implies the transfer of the copyright from the author to the publisher upon acceptance. Accepted papers become the permanent property of 'Acta Haematologica' and may not be reproduced by any means, in whole or in part, without the written consent of the publisher. It is the author's responsibility to obtain permission to reproduce illustrations, tables, etc. from other publications.

Arrangement:

Recommendation for Usage of Units and Abbreviations: The Editorial Board of 'Acta Haematologica' supports the recommendations of the 'International Committee for Standardization in Hematology' for using the SI (Système International d'Unités) equivalents in haematological literature. The standard abbreviations used for measurements of weight, length, volume, and time (i.e., mg, cm, ml, min) are used without definition. The abbreviations listed below also require no preliminary definition. Please note that punctuation is not needed. When using other abbreviations, spell out the name in full at the first mention, and follow with the abbreviation in parentheses.

Title page: The first page of each paper should indicate the title (main title underlined), the authors' names, and the institute where the work was conducted. A short title for use as running head is also required.

Key words: For indexing purposes, a list of 3 – 10 key words in English is essential.

Abstract: Each paper needs an abstract of up to 10 lines.

Small type: Paragraphs which can or must be set in smaller type (case histories, test methods, etc.) should be indicated with a 'p' (petit) in the margin on the left-hand side.

Footnotes: Avoid footnotes. When essential, they are numbered consecutively and typed at the foot of the appropriate page.

Tables and illustrations: Tables and illustrations (both numbered in Arabic numerals) should be prepared on separate sheets. Tables require a heading and figures a legend, also prepared on a separate sheet. For the reproduction of illustrations, only good drawings and original photographs can be accepted; negatives or photocopies cannot be used. When possible, group several illustrations on one block for reproduction (max. size 176 × 224 mm) or provide crop marks. On the back of each illustration, indicate its number, the author's name, and 'top'. Color illustrations are reproduced at the author's expense.

References: In the text identify references by Arabic numerals [in square brackets]. Material submitted for publication but not yet accepted should be noted as 'unpublished data' and not be included in the reference list. The list of references should include only those publications which are cited in the text. Do not alphabetize; number references in the order in which they are first mentioned in the text. The surnames of the authors followed by initials should be given. There should be no punctuation other than a comma to separate the authors. Cite all authors, 'et al' is not sufficient. Abbreviate journal names according to the Index Medicus system. (Also see International Committee of Medical Journal Editors: Uniform requirements for manuscripts submitted to biomedical journals. Br Med J 1988;296:401–405.)

Examples

(a) Papers published in periodicals: Kauffman HF, van der Heide S, Beaumont F, Blok H, de Vries K: Class-specific antibody determination against *Aspergillus fumigatus* by means of the enzyme-linked immunosorbent assay. III. Comparative study: IgG, IgA, IgM ELISA titers, precipitating antibodies and IgE binding after fractionation of the antigen. Int Arch Allergy Appl Immunol 1986;80:300–306.

(b) Monographs: Matthews DE, Farewell VT: Using and Understanding Medical Statistics. Basel, Karger, 1985.

(c) Edited books: Hardy WD Jr, Essex M: FeLV-induced feline acquired immune deficiency syndrome: A model for human AIDS; in Klein E (ed): Acquired Immunodeficiency Syndrome. Prog Allergy. Basel, Karger, 1986, vol 37, pp 353–376.

Full address: The exact postal address complete with postal code of the senior author must be given. If correspondence is handled by someone else, indicate this accordingly.

Further details: Authors may consult our leaflet 'Rules for the Preparation of Manuscripts', available on request from the Publisher, S. Karger AG, P.O. Box, CH – 4009 Basel (Switzerland).

Page charges: Authors are charged SFr. 115.– / US $ 75.00 per printed page for the first 6 pages and SFr. 225.– / US $ 150.00 for each additional page, including tables, illustrations, and references. 1 printed page is equal to approximately 3 manuscript pages.

Galley proofs: Unless indicated otherwise, galley proofs are sent to the first-named author and should be returned with the least possible delay. Alterations made in galley proofs, other than the correction of printer's errors, are charged to the author. No page proofs are supplied.

Reprints: Order forms and a price list are sent with the galley proofs. Orders submitted after the issue is printed are subject to considerably higher prices. Allow five weeks from date of publication for delivery of reprints.

Entity	Abbreviation	Recommended SI equivalent	Not recommended
Red blood cell count	RBC	10^{12}/l	10^{6}/mm^{3}
White blood cell count	WBC	10^{9}/l	10^{3}/mm^{3}
Platelet count		... × 10^{9}/l	... × 10^{3}/mm^{3}
Reticulocyte count		% (or ... × 10^{9}/l)	‰ (or ../mm^{3})
Haemoglobin	Hb	g/dl[a]	g/100 ml
Packed cell volume	PCV	ratio[b]	%
Mean cell volume	MCV	fl	
Mean cell haemoglobin	MCH	pg	
Mean cell haemoglobin concentration	MCHC	g/dl	%
Mean cell diameter	MCD	µm	
Sedimentation rate	ESR	mm in 1 h[c]	
Plasma haemoglobin	Plasma Hb	mg/l	mg/100 ml
Serum vitamin B_{12}		ng/l	
Serum folate		µg/l	
Serum iron		µmol/l	µg/100 ml
Total iron binding capacity	TIBC	µmol/l	µg/100 ml
Unsaturated iron binding capacity	UIBC	µmol/l	µg/100 ml
Transferrin		g/l	mg/100 ml
Serum haptoglobin		g/l	mg/100 ml
Plasma fibrinogen		g/l	mg/100 ml

[a] The concentration for Hb only is expressed as ../dl and not ../l or ../100 ml.

[b] No unit necessary, 1/1 is implied.

[c] Indicate method only if other than Westergren.

KARGER

Supplement Issue
Included in subscription

Chemotherapy (ISSN 0009–3157), **Vol. 37, Suppl. 1 (1991)**
Editor: Hans Schönfeld, Grenzach

Editor: Kihachiro Shimizu, Tokyo

Ofloxacin in Compromised Host

International Ofloxacin Symposium
Vancouver, Canada, July 12, 1990

Quinolones, new potent antimicrobial agents which are particularly effective in intractable infections such as those frequently seen in compromised hosts, are the focus of this supplement issue. Contributed by internationally recognized experts, the papers report and discuss the mechanism of action of new quinolones in general and ofloxacin in particular. The papers demonstrate the ease-of-use and high efficacy of ofloxacin in therapy, which open new fields for the use of oral anti-bacterials in severe infections in compromised hosts. The issue provides stimulating reading for specialists in the clinical treatment of infectious diseases and for those involved in research on new quinolones per se.

Contents

Shimizu, K.: Introduction
Smith, J.T.: Ofloxacin, a Bactericidal Antibacterial
Yamaoka, M.; Fukuchi, Y.; Yokouchi, M. et al.: Efficacy of Oral Administration of Ofloxacin in Lower Respiratory Tract Infections in Aged Patients with Chronic Lung Disease
Giamarellou, H.; Iakovou, M.; Pistoni, M. et al.: Kinetics and Comparative Efficacy of Ofloxacin versus Co-Trimoxazole in the Asymptomatic Bacteriuria of Elderly Subjects
Sawada, H.; Tashima, M.; Okuma, M.: Use of Ofloxacin in Prevention and Treatment of Secondary Infections in Hematological Malignancies
Gluckman, E.; Roudet, C.; Hirsch, I. et al.: Prophylaxis of Bacterial Infections after Bone Marrow Transplantation. A Randomized Prospective Study Comparing Oral Broad-Spectrum Nonabsorbable Antibiotics (Vancomycin-Tobramycin-Colistin) to Absorbable Antibiotics (Ofloxacin-Amoxicillin)
De Simone, C.; Di Fabio, S.; Moretti, S. et al.: Open Randomized Controlled Parallel Study of Ofloxacin versus Trimethoprim-Sulfamethoxazole Treatment of Lower Respiratory Tract and Urinary Infections
Nicolle, L.E.; Degelau, J.; Alessi, P. et al.: Ofloxacin Use in a Geriatric Population
Sato, A.; Shichi, I.; Iwata, M. et al.: Long Term Effects of Ofloxacin on Clinical Courses in Patients with Diffuse Panbronchiolitis.
Matsumoto, T.; Kumazawa, J.; Ueda, S. et al.: Treatment of Complicated Urinary Tract Infections with Ofloxacin following an Aminoglycoside
Rubinstein, E.: International Ofloxacin Symposium – Closing Remarks

Fields of Interest
Pharmacology, Infectious Diseases

Chemotherapy, Vol. 37, Suppl. 1 (1991)
Ofloxacin in Compromised Host
International Ofloxacin Symposium
Vancouver, Canada, July 12, 1990
Editor: Shimizu, K. (Tokyo)
IV + 72 p., 15 fig., 1 cpl., 32 tab., soft cover, 1991
SFr. 58.– / DM 69.– / £ 25.30 / US $ 46.50
US $ price for USA, £ price for UK only (subject to change)
ISBN 3–8055–5423–0

KARGER

KI 91084

Haematopoietic Growth Factors: Biology and Clinical Use

Editor:
Elio E. Polli, Milano

8 figures and 9 tables, 1991

KARGER

S. Karger · Medical and Scientific Publishers
Basel · München · Paris · London · New York · New Delhi · Bangkok · Singapore · Tokyo · Sydney

Drug Dosage

The authors and the publisher have exerted every effort to ensure that drug selection and dosage set forth in this text are in accord with current recommendations and practice at the time of publication. However, in view of ongoing research, changes in government regulations, and the constant flow of information relating to drug therapy and drug reactions, the reader is urged to check the package insert for each drug for any change in indications and dosage and for added warnings and precautions. This is particularly important when the recommended agent is a new and/or infrequently employed drug.

Printed in Switzerland on acid-free paper by
Buchdruckerei Basler Zeitung, Basel
ISBN 3–8055–5557–1

Contents

Introduction
Polli, E.E. 121

In vitro Biological Activities of the Haemopoietic Growth Factors: Implications for Their Clinical Use
Testa, N.G. 122

Hematopoietic Growth Factors: Interactions and Regulation of Production
Brach, M.A.; Herrmann, F. 128

Clinical Role of Colony Stimulating Factors
Brugger, W.; Rosenthal, F.M.; Kanz, L.; Mertelsmann, R. 138

The Role of Interleukin-1 in Hematopoiesis
Fibbe, W.E.; Willemze, R. 148

The Role of Haematopoietic Growth Factors in Bone Marrow Transplantation
Polli, E.E. 155

Erythropoietin: Clinical Applications
Foa, P. 162

Introduction

Acta Haematol 1991;86:121

Haematopoietic growth factors (HGFs) are a family of glycoproteins regulating proliferation, differentiation and function of the haematopoietic cell lineages.

In the last few years, our understanding of the biology of HGFs has tremendously increased. Moreover, several of these molecules have been isolated and are now being produced by recombinant DNA techniques.

Undoubtedly, the availability of biosynthetic HGFs for clinical purposes represents one of the most interesting and promising achievements not only for modern haematology, but also for other strictly related disciplines, as for instance immunology and oncology.

Several HGFs as erythropoietin, granulocyte colony-stimulating factor, granulocyte-macrophage colony-stimulating factor and interleukin-3, are already being tested in patients with a variety of clinical conditions requiring an enhancement of haematopoietic proliferation and/or differentiation and/or function.

Results so far achieved not only have opened innovative therapeutic perspectives, but have also contributed to widen our understanding of the physiopathology of haematopoiesis.

This issue of *Acta Haematologica* attempts to provide an updated and critical view at the main biological and clinical aspects of some of the HGFs which are presently under investigation for therapeutic use.

E.E. Polli

Acta Haematol 1991;86:122–127

0001–5792/91/0863–0122 $2.75/0

In vitro Biological Activities of the Haemopoietic Growth Factors: Implications for Their Clinical Use

N.G. Testa

Paterson Institute for Cancer Research, Christie Hospital, Manchester, UK

Key Words. Cell proliferation · Colony-stimulating factors · Differentiation · Interleukin 3

Abstract. The recent availability of several haemopoietic growth factors in purified recombinant form suitable for clinical use has prompted their use in haematology and oncology. The knowledge of their various effects in vitro on cell proliferation, differentiation and function and of their target cell populations will help in the design of treatment protocols with regard to selcction of the best growth factor (or combination of them) for specific desired effects.

Introduction

The roles of the haemopoietic growth factors were first elucidated using in vitro techniques, and only later was their physiological significance assayed in vivo. Indeed, with the exception of erythropoietin, these factors were first detected using in vitro techniques after a long and unrewarding search in in vivo systems. The purification and the eventual availability of growth factors in recombinant form has also been crucially helped by the use of in vitro testing of their activities.

The reductionist approach using highly purified populations of haemopoietic progenitors (colony-forming cells, CFC, with the ability to proliferate and develop in soft gels in culture, giving rise to clonal colonies containing mature cells) stimulated with purified growth factors yields valuable information on the direct action of single factors on discrete cell populations. Stimulation with combinations of factors allows the investigation of additive, potentiating or inhibitory effects on cellular proliferation, as well as on the selection of the lineage of differentiation by multipotential cells. In contrast, the study of unpurified cell populations from the bone marrow allows the study of cell-cell interactions and of secondary effects attributable to cascade-type phenomena due to the secondary production of growth factors (and other bioregulators) by accessory cells. These regulatory cells may be of lymphohaemopoietic origin (i.e. macrophages or T cells) or be part of the bone marrow stroma.

In this review, we will highlight the applications of in vitro systems not only for increasing our basic understanding of the regulation of cell proliferation and differentiation in haemopoiesis, but also in the logical planning of the clinical applications of growth factors discussed elsewhere in this volume.

Effect of Growth Factors on Cell Proliferation and Differentiation

Effects on Proliferation

The mandatory role of growth factors in promoting the proliferation of CFC is the property that allowed first their detection and subsequently their characterisation, and led to the name of colony-stimulating factors (CSF) that is still used for some of them. However, it later became apparent that they have a multiplicity of roles: they influence cell survival in vitro

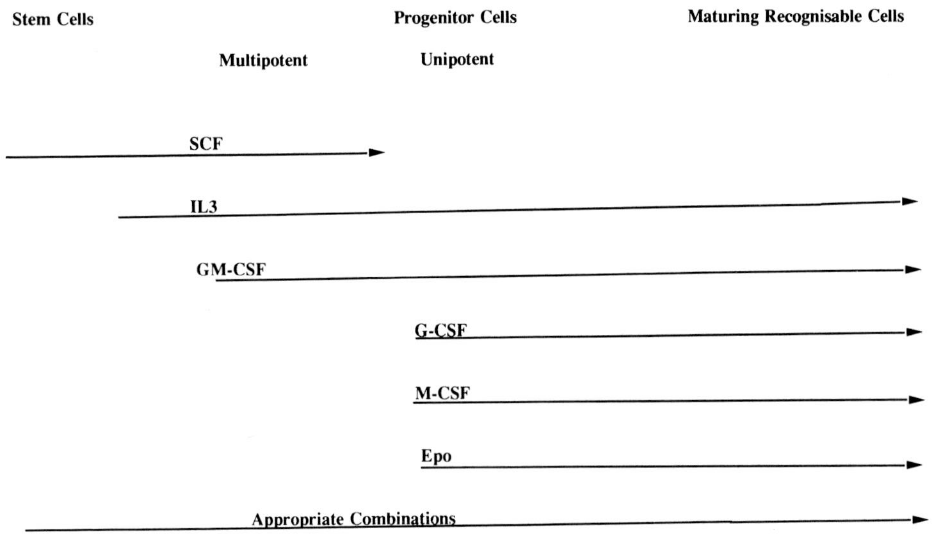

Fig. 1. Range of target cells for the haemopoietic growth factor. SCF = stem cell factor; Epo = erythropoietin.

and cellular differentiation and induce or enhance the functional activity of the mature cells. The ability of CSF to stimulate the proliferation and development of haemopoietic progenitors allowed their characterisation as a functional group of molecules, a concept validated later by the interactions demonstrated between their specific receptors, the influence of one factor on the rate of production of another, and the suggestion of some common signalling pathways [reviewed by Metcalf, 1988].

The heterogeneity of the CSF and the lack of any significant homology within the group suggest that they are not derived from a common ancestral gene. Despite this, there is considerable overlap in their target cells, a fact demonstrated by the functional detection of specific receptors for more than one factor (maybe for all of the CSF) in cells from populations highly enriched for primitive CFC [Heyworth et al., 1988] and also in the recognisable cells in the bone marrow [Nicola, 1990]. These findings indicate a high level of redundancy in the system for reasons which are not yet clear, although it is logical to expect that this redundancy may play a role in the fine adjustment of both cell proliferation and cell differentiation. For example, murine cell populations highly enriched for primitive CFC respond to interleukin 3 (IL-3), producing large numbers of colonies, but only a small proportion of the cells with the capacity to respond to IL-3 will respond to granulocyte CSF (G-CSF) or macrophage CSF (M-CSF) with colony formation. However, these two factors acting together have a synergistic effect on the numbers of colonies produced by stimulating the CFC which cannot respond to either factor acting alone (fig. 1). Thus, cells not able to respond to one factor in isolation may respond to combinations of factors, several of which have been shown to have more than additive effects [Heyworth et al., 1988]. Synergistic effects have also been described in human CFC [McNiece et al., 1989]. As the target cells were, as mentioned above, highly purified, it is likely that the effects observed were direct effects on the CFC. Also, as the factors are required to be present from the initiation of the cultures, one implication is that the primitive CSF have receptors for many, if not all, of the growth factors from early stages of development. This is an important concept for the rational planning of clinical trials.

Effects on Differentiation

Another important point is that the balance of growth factors to which a cell is exposed may determine the lineage(s) of differentiation (table 1). Thus, IL-3 will stimulate all the myeloid lineages and granulocyte-macrophage CSF (GM-CSF) the majority of them (although it may recruit fewer of the multipotential progenitors than IL-3; fig. 1). In contrast, the more lineage-restricted factors G- and M-CSF and erythropoietin will preferentially stimulate the late progenitor cells which may be already committed to a specific cell lineage and will produce the mature progeny of that lineage (table 2). When factors are used in combination, not only the range of target cells is increased, but the cell lineage(s) stimulated may be different. Thus, the CFC which respond to IL-3 pro-

Table 1. Growth factors and their target cells

Target colony forming cells	Growth factors						
	SCF	IL3	GM-CSF	G-CSF	M-CSF	IL5	Epo
Blast-CFC	+	+	+	–	–	–	–
Mix-CFC	+	+	+	–	–	–	–
GM-CFC		+	+	+	+	–	–
G-CFC		+	+	+	±[1]	–	–
M-CFC		+	+	±[1]	+	–	–
Eo-CFC		+	+	–	–	+	–
Meg-CFC		+	+	–	–	–	?
Ba-CFC		+	–	–	–	–	–
BFU-E	+	+	+	–	–	–	±
CFU-E		–	–	–	–	–	+

Mix = mixed; Eo = eosinophilic; Meg = megakaryocyte; Ba = basophil; BFU-E = early erythroid progenitor, burst-forming unit, erythroid; CFU-E = late erythroid progenitor, colony-forming unit, erythroid; SCF = stem cell factor; Epo = erythropoietin.
[1] Only at high concentrations.

Table 2. Haemopoietic growth factors

Name	Major types of cells produced in vitro
IL-3	neutrophilic granulocytes, monocyte-macrophages, eosinophils, basophils and mast cells; erythrocytes (if erythropoietin also present); megakaryocytes
GM-CSF	granulocytes, monocyte-macrophages, eosinophils, megakaryocytes
G-CSF	neutrophilic granulocytes, monocyte-macrophages (at high concentrations)
M-CSF	macrophages, neutrophilic granulocytes (at high concentrations)
IL-5	eosinophils
Erythropoietin	erythrocytes

Table 3. Cycling status of GM-CFC after in vivo G-CSF

	Day 0	Day 5
Percent in S phase	55 ± 13	63 ± 11
Number of patients	9	6

Data calculated from Bronchud et al. [1988].

ducing several myeloid lineages will respond to G-CSF + M-CSF producing only neutrophils and macrophages, or to interleukin 1 (IL-1) (which has no colony-stimulating activity) + M-CSF with the production of macrophages. Dramatic synergies were also observed between G-CSF and GM-CSF [Heyworth et al., 1988].

These data imply that the potential lineage of differentiation is not a predetermined and intrinsic property of primitive progenitor cells, but may be determined by the balance of factors present in the adjacent cellular environment. Those factors include not only the haemopoietic growth factors, but other cytokines like IL-1, that can modulate colony formation acting in conjunction with growth factors, but which have no colony-stimulating activity of their own.

It can be seen from figure 1 that factors like IL-3 and the recently described stem cell factor [Whitte, 1990] act on the more primitive haemopoietic cells. Both may need to act together with other factors to stimulate maximum production of mature cells, and the relative levels of each factor may favour different developmental behaviour. Thus, it is known that high levels of IL-3 favour self-reproduction at the expense of differentiation in murine stem cell lines: these cells kept in high levels of IL-3 self-reproduce but do not produce clonogenic cells which may respond to G- or GM-CSF [Heyworth et al., 1990]. Low levels of IL-3 favour differentiation when acting together with G- or GM-CSF, while intermediate levels of IL-3 result in an equilibrium between self-renewal and differentiation. One possible mechanism for these effects is that IL-3 at high concentrations down-modulates GM- and G-CSF receptors [Walker et al., 1985], thus favouring self-renewal over differentiation. It is therefore reasonable to expect that sequential use of IL-3 followed by GM- or G-CSF will potentiate the effect of the latter if the IL-3 has generated more target cells on which the other factors may act. In fact, such data are beginning to emerge, both from experimental animals and from clinical trials discussed elsewhere in this issue.

The more lineage-restricted growth factors may act mainly (or solely) expanding the post-CFC maturing cell compartment. This was clearly indicated by data obtained from patients treated with G-CSF [Bronchud et al., 1988]: bone marrow cultured after 5 days of treatment with doses which induced neutrophilia showed practically no change in the proportion of GM-CFC undergoing DNA synthesis (table 3). Another indication that the progenitor cell compartment is little influenced by this factor is the stability of the ratio GM-CFC to BFU-E (burst-forming unit-erythroid) in the bone marrow, while the ratio of recognisable myeloid to erythroid cells more than doubles (table 4). This is taken as an indication that the increase in the numbers of neutrophilic granulocytes observed after treatment with G-CSF is due to stimulation of the post-CFC compartment, a concept also supported by the shortening of the cell cycle times in the maturing myeloid cells [Lord et al., 1989]. These observations pointing to a target population placed relatively late in the myeloid maturation pathway make G-CSF a factor of choice when a quick neutrophilia is desired.

Growth Factors and Mature Cell Function

There is a vast range of functional activities required to regulate the host response to infection that can be induced or enhanced by growth factors in mature myeloid cells (table 5) [Gough and Nicola, 1990; Nicola, 1990; Devereux et al., 1989]. These observations give a logical base for the use of CSF for the treatment of patients with life-threatening infections, or as preventive treatment in high-risk patients. The usefulness of G-CSF in preventing infection after chemotherapy has already been demonstrated [Bronchud et al., 1988], and it is reasonable to expect extension of this treatment for example to patients with extensive burns or with exposed fractures. The effects on mature cells also support a role for G- and GM-CSF when defective cell production is accompanied by abnormal function of the mature cells, like in myelodysplasia, as discussed elsewhere in this issue.

Growth Factors and Stem Cells

The regulation of stem cell renewal (to maintain their numbers in steady state and to replenish the population after cytotoxic injury or following bone marrow transplantation) takes place within the bone marrow microenvironment through processes which are not yet completely understood. Stromal cells and

Table 4. Myeloid/erythroid ratios after in vivo G-CSF

	Day 0	Day 5
GM-CFC/BFU-E	2.2 ± 0.3	2.6 ± 0.2
Myeloid/erythroid bone marrow cells	4.2 ± 0.2	9.2 ± 1.7[1]

Data calculated from Bronchud et al. [1988].
[1] Significantly different.

Table 5. Effects of CSF on mature cells

Factor	Target cells	
G-CSF	neutrophils	↑ antibody-dependent cell-mediated cytotoxicity
		↑ generation of superoxide anion
		↑ release of arachidonic acid in response to chemoattractants
GM-CSF	neutrophils	↑ priming of cells to activation by bacterial protein
		↑ antibody-dependent cell-mediated cytotoxicity
		↑ metabolic energy
		↑ phagocytosis (bacteria, parasites, yeast), inhibits migration
		↑ cell adhesiveness to endothelium
		↑ generation of superoxide
		↑ production of IL1
	monocytes	↑ chemotaxis
		↑ release of prostaglandin E, plasminogen activator, interferons, tumour necrosis factor, M-CSF
		↑ antibody-dependent cytotoxicity
		↑ cell adhesion

Table 6. Effect of the addition of G-CSF or IL-3 to long-term cultures

	Increase in GM-CFC		
	supernatant	adherent layer	optimum time
G-CSF	<2×	2.2×	3–4 weeks
IL3	5–6×	8.5×	3–4 weeks

Data calculated from Coutinho et al. [1990].

their secreted or membrane-bound regulatory factors form permissive or inductive microenvironments in which self-renewal or differentiation may preferentially take place [Lord and Testa, 1989].

One possibility to ponder in the initial days of the clinical trials was whether the stimulation of the haemopoietic system, especially when the complement of stem cells was expected to be low, could lead to eventual exhaustion and to secondary hypoplasia. As discussed above, this risk appears to be negligible in the case of the more lineage-specific growth factors, which would have little direct influence on the stem cells. Some data on long-term bone marrow cultures treated with high doses of CSF for the whole culture periods of several weeks showed that the effect on progenitor cells (table 6) and also on total cell production was transient and did not lead to a shortening of the life-span of the cultures, as would be expected if the stem cells had been exhaused [Coutinho et al., 1990]. This was the case even for IL-3-treated cultures where the most marked expansion in GM-CFC was observed (table 6). However, the effect of combinations of factors that may alter the balance between self-reproduction and differentiation remains to be explored.

The experimental and clinical evidence available indicates that correction of a stem cell defect, for example in aplastic anaemia or, in chemotherapy-treated patients, with expansion of the stem cell compartment to normal levels will not be achieved with the myeloid growth factors. Even if those factors heighten mature cell production and ameliorate the clinical syndrome, it is difficult at present to envisage a cure [Testa and Dexter, 1990].

However, this might be achieved with other factors. The stem cell factor recently described [Whitte, 1990] influences migration and proliferation of stem cells and of melanocyte stem cells, as well as of haemopoietic stem cells. This factor is produced by stromal cells in the bone marrow and is likely to be an important regulator of stem cell renewal and proliferation. It can exist as a free or membrane-bound molecule and may thus act by cell-to-cell interaction. It may also potentiate the proliferative effects of other factors on primitive haemopoietic cells [Zsebo et al., 1990]. Its possible role on the expansion of the stem cell population is the subject of intense interest at present. However, optimum production of mature cells may still require the administration of the myeloid growth factors.

Other factors, originally described as regulators of B cells, like IL-4 and IL-6, have been shown to have a stimulatory effect on multipotential cells in the bone marrow [Kishi et al., 1989; Heyworth et al., 1988; Ikebuchi et al., 1988] and are, at present, undergoing the first clinical trials.

General Comments

The knowledge of fundamental steps in cell development opened the possibility of the logical manipulation of cell production in therapy. The first clear indication was the use of erythropoietin as replacement therapy to correct the anaemia of renal disease, an indication proposed many years before the recombinant molecule became available for clinical use. Up to now, hundreds of patients have been treated with erythropoietin with outstanding success.

The clinical trials discussed elsewhere in this volume already show clear indications for the use of myeloid growth factors in therapy. Based on the in vitro data, logical choices about finer manipulation of the haemopoietic system, both with regard to increased cell output and to the desired lineages to be stimulated, can be contemplated. The use of combinations of factors appears particularly interesting, and this will allow the fine manipulation of the system to obtain expansion of the desired cell populations and a better timing of the response. This will also exploit the use of the superadditive effects of some combinations of factors and lead to reductions of the therapeutic doses. It is already clear that we can manipulate the production of mature cells in patients. Manipulation of the stem cell population (for example to correct aplastic anaemia, or to expand the stem cells in vitro for use in transplantation) is the next desirable development.

References

Bronchud MH, Potter MR, Morgenstern G, Blasco MJ, Scarffe JH, Thatcher N, Crowther D, Souza LM, Alton NK, Testa NG, Dexter TM: In vitro and in vivo analysis of the effects of recombinant human granulocyte colony-stimulating factor in patients. Br J Cancer 1988;58:64–69.

Coutinho L, Will A, Radford J, Schiro R, Testa NG, Dexter TM: Effects of recombinant human granulocyte colony-stimulating factor (CSF), human granulocyte macrophage-CSF and gibbon interleukin-3 on hematopoiesis in human long-term bone marrow culture. Blood 1990;75:2118–2129.

Devereux S, Bull HA, Campos-Costa D, Sails R, Linch DC: Granulocyte-macrophage colony stimulating factor induced changes in cellular adhesion molecular expression and adhesion to endothelium: In vitro and in vivo studies in man. Br J Haematol 1989;71:323–330.

Gough NM, Nicola NA: Granulocyte-macrophage colony stimulating factors; in Dexter TM, Garland J, Testa NG (eds): Colony Stimulating Factors: Cellular and Molecular Biology. New York, Dekker, 1990, pp 111–153.

Heyworth CM, Dexter TM, Kan O, Whetton AD: The role of hemopoietic growth factors in self-renewal and differentiation of IL-3-dependent multipotential stem cells. Growth Factors 1990;2:197–211.

Heyworth CM, Ponting ILO, Dexter TM: The response of haemopoietic cells to growth factors: Developmental implications of synergistic interactions. J Cell Sci 1988;91:239–247.

Ikebuchi K, Ihle JN, Hirai Y, Wong GG, Clark SC, Ogawa M: Synergistic factors for stem cell proliferation. Further studies on the target stem cells and the mechanism of stimulation by interleukin-1, interleukin-6 and granulocyte-colony stimulating factor. Blood 1988;72:2007–2014.

Kishi K, Ihle JN, Undal DL, Ogawa M: Murine B-cell stimulatory factor-1 (BSF-1)/Interleukin-4 (IL-4) is a multilineage colony-stimulating factor that acts directly on primitive haemopoietic progenitors. J Cell Physiol 1989;139:463–468.

Lord BI, Bronchud MH, Owens S, Chang J, Howell A, Souza L, Dexter TM: The kinetics of human granulopoiesis following treatment with granulocyte colony-stimulating factor in vivo. Proc Natl Acad Sci USA 1989;86:9499–9503.

Lord BI, Testa NG: The hemopoietic system: Structure and regulation; in Testa NG, Gale RP (eds): Hematopoiesis: Long-Term Effects of Chemotherapy and Radiation. New York, Dekker, 1989, pp 1–26.

McNiece I, Andrews R, Stewart M, Clark S, Boone T, Quesenberry P: Action of interleukin 3, G-CSF and GM-CSF on highly enriched human hematopoietic progenitor cells: Synergistic interactions of GM-CSF plus G-CSF. Blood 1989;74:110–114.

Metcalf D: The molecular control of blood cells. Cambridge, Harvard University Press, 1988.

Nicola NA: Granulocyte colony-stimulating factor; in Dexter TM, Garland J, Testa NG (eds): Colony Stimulating Factors: Molecular and Cellular Biology. New York, Dekker, 1990, pp 77–109.

Testa NG, Dexter TM: Haemopoietic growth factors and haematological malignancies. Clin Endocrinol Metabol 1990;4:177–189.

Walker F, Nicola NA, Metcalf D, Burgess AW: Hierarchical downmodulation of hemopoietic growth factor receptors. Cell 1985;43:269–276.

Whitte ON: Steel locus defines new multipotent growth factors. Cell 1990;63:5–6.

Zsebo KM, Williams DA, Geissler EN, Broudy VC, Martin FH, Atkins HL, Hsu RY, Birkett NC, Okino KH, Murdock DC, Jacobsen FW, Pangley KE, Smith KA, Takeishi T, Cattanach BM, Galli SJ, Suggs SV: Stem cell factor is encoded at the Sl locus of the mouse and is the ligand for the c-kit tyrosine kinase receptor. Cell 1990;63:213–224.

N.G. Testa, MD, PhD
Paterson Institute for Cancer Research
Christie Hospital
Manchester M20 9BY (UK)

Acta Haematol 1991;86:128–137

0001–5792/91/0863–0128 $ 2.75/0

Hematopoietic Growth Factors: Interactions and Regulation of Production

Marion A. Brach, Friedhelm Herrmann

Department of Internal Medicine I (Hematology and Oncology), University of Freiburg Medical Center, Freiburg, FRG

Key Words. Colony-stimulating factors · CSF gene regulation · Cytokine network · Cytokine signal-transduction

Abstract. Hematopoietic growth factors are the major regulatory molecules supporting constitutive and inducible hematopoiesis. Molecular biology techniques have led to the identification and cloning of a series of hematopoietic growth factor genes, and the synthesis of large amounts of these molecules has facilitated investigations or their physiological functions and the network of their interactions. The present article focuses on the role of hematopoietic growth factors, growth-factor-synergizing factors, and growth-factor-releasing factors in the regulation of proliferation, differentiation, and functional activation of hematopoietic stem cells and lineage-committed progenitor cells. Cellular sources of growth factors, signal transduction pathways involved in their gene activation and transcriptional and posttranscriptional mechanisms that govern regulation of expression of these genes are also detailed.

Introduction

Hormone-like polypeptides termed colony-stimulating factors (CSFs) regulate the proliferation and differentiation of hematopoietic cells by establishing a complex network of interacting and interdependent stimulatory and inhibitory loops that ensure homeostatic blood cell production during steady-state hematopoiesis but also adapt the levels of circulating blood cells to situations of increased need of functional end cells during inducible hematopoiesis. Intense research over the past years has not only elucidated the specific functions of single CSFs, but has also shown that a variety of their effects are achieved by synergistic cooperation of different CSFs or related molecules. Unlike with classic hormones, CSF production is not restricted to specific sites or specific cell types, but CSFs are secreted by various cell types common to most organs. Cellular sources of CSFs include T cells, NK cells, B cells, granulocytes, monocytes as well as mesenchymal cells such as vascular endothelial cells, smooth muscle cells and fibroblasts [see ref. 38 for review]. Stimuli that induce CSF synthesis relate to a wide range of physiological and nonphysiological signals, including cytokines themselves, agonists of various signal transduction pathways, several tumor-promoting phorbol compounds, DNA-damaging agents such as arabinofuranosylcytosine, or ionizing irradiation [see ref. 1 for review]. Molecular biology techniques have led to the identification of the structure of most of the CSF genes. Despite several differences, features common to the regulation of the expression of most of the hematopoietic cytokine genes became evident such as cis-acting elements in promoter regions, allowing coordinated activation of the respective genes. In addition, similarities in the 3′untranslated regions of the CSF genes that predispose their transcripts to rapid turnover, and thus ensure tight posttranscriptional control, have been identified. We review the biological activities of various hematopoietic growth factors, signal transduction pathways leading to their synthesis and the transcriptional and posttranscriptional regulatory mechanisms that govern the expression of their genes.

Role of Growth Factors in Hematopoiesis

Blood cells in circulation have a very short life span ranging from a few hours to several weeks. Proliferation and differentiation of multipotent stem cells located in the bone marrow ensure a continuous supply of blood cells and thus maintain levels of circulating cells within a narrow range. Stem cells have the capacity to self-renew and to undergo differentiation into progenitor cells which are then subjected to lineage-committed terminal divisions. Survival, proliferation, and functional maturation of the various hematopoietic cells are regulated in vitro by a network of interdependent hematopoietic growth factors [17, 22]. Studies over the past years have indicated that both steady-state and inducible hematopoiesis are regulated by distinct pathways. Constitutive hematopoiesis ensures steady-state levels of blood cells, while inducible hematopoiesis is required to adapt levels of circulating blood cells to situations of increased demand of the respective end cells, for instance under conditions of inflammatory responses, infections or hemorrhage. Steady-state hematopoiesis is regulated by the constitutive release of macrophage (M)- and granulocyte (G)-CSF by fibroblasts [60, 72] and perhaps more importantly by the recently identified stem cell factor (SCF), also referred to as kit-ligand [see ref. 111 for a review]. SCF exerts multiple effects on various hematopoietic subpopulations but requires the cooperation with colony-stimulating factors for optimum stimulatory effects. In contrast, inducible hematopoiesis is initiated by a cascade of cytokines secreted from T cells and monocytes in response to various stimuli (fig. 1). Upon exposure to antigen, T cells release interleukin (IL)-2 [69], IL-4 [52], IL-5 [29, 90], IL-6 [41] and tumor necrosis factor alpha (TNFα) [8]. IL-2 autostimulates T cells to synthesize GM-CSF, and IL-3 [76]. Activated monocytes release IL-1 [109], G-CSF [77], M-CSF [42], IL-6 [10], IL-7 and IL-9 [40] to spur proliferation and functional maturation of respective lineage-committed progenitor cells. Recent studies have also demonstrated that endothelial cells stimulated by IL-1 or TNFα secrete numerous cytokines and thus take part in the complex scenario of inducible hematopoiesis [15, 93, 100] (fig. 2). In addition, bacterial endotoxins and various virus-encoded proteins are potent inducers of cytokine synthesis by mesenchymal cells, T cells and monocytes [9, 23, 64, 83, 106]. Table 1 gives an overview of the various polypeptides regulating hematopoiesis, describes the cellular sources of these molecules, their molecular weights, chromosomal locations and mode of secretion.

The biological specificities of the various hematopoietic growth factors are complex, overlapping and for the most part redundant. According to their capacity to target distinct hematopoietic cell subsets, these polypeptides can be classified into several categories. Hematopoietic growth factors per se include the colony-stimulating factors which act directly on various hematopoietic subpopulations and encompass G-, M-, GM-CSF, erythropoietin (EPO), IL-3 (also

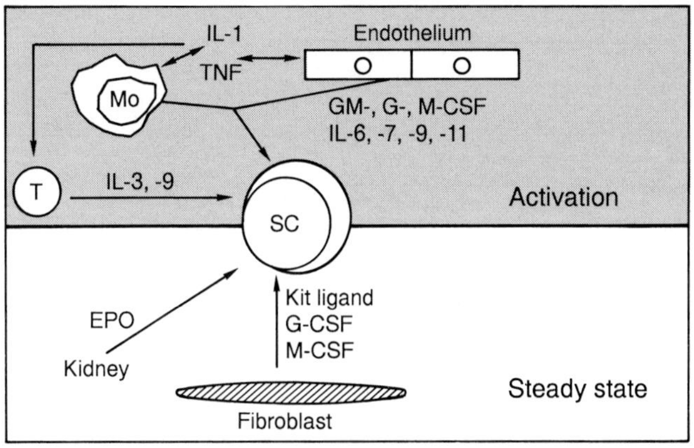

Fig. 1. Interactions of hematopoietic cytokines in steady state and inducible hematopoiesis. For abbrevations see text.

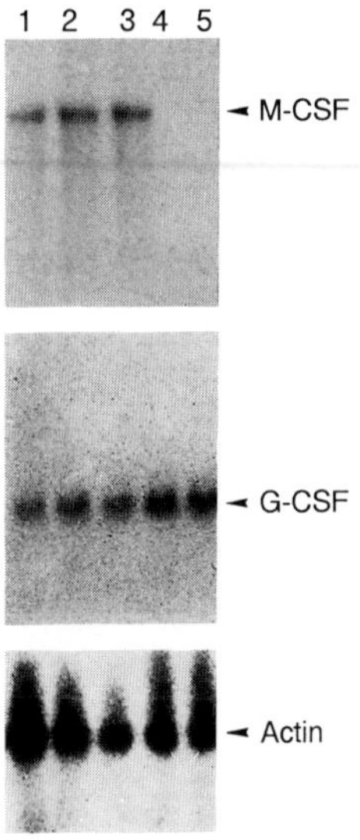

Fig. 2. mRNA accumulation of M-CSF and G-CSF by neutrophils (lane 1), monocytes (lane 2), and fibroblasts (lane 3). Cells were treated for 18 h with recombinant human GM-CSF (25 ng/ml) prior to RNA extraction. Lane 4 represents RNA obtained from circulating blood cells of a patient with stable-phase chronic myelogenous leukemia. In lane 6, cytoplasmatic RNA of a patient with acute myelogenous leukemia was hybridized with M-CSF and G-CSF specific cDNA probes. Hybridization with an α-actin cDNA compares RNA loading in single lanes.

Table 1. Cytokines involved in the regulation of hematopoiesis

Molecule	Synonym	Chromos. localisat.	mRNA kb	MW, kD	Secretion[1]	Main source[2]
Hematopoietic growth factors						
SCF	MGF, kit-ligand	nr	nr	18	p	F, hepatoma
multi-CSF	IL-3	5q	1	14–18	p	T
GM-CSF	CSF-α	5q21-32	1	14–35	e; p	T, E, F
G-CSF	CSF-β	17q11-22	1.6	18–22	e; p	M, G, E, F
M-CSF	CSF-1	5q33	1.8–4.0	36–90	e; a	M, G, E, F
Erythropoietin		7q21	2.0	32–35	p	kidney
Non-CSF interleukins						
IL-1-α	hemopoietin-1	2q14	2.2	17–31	e; p; a	M, G, E, F
IL-1-β		2q14	1.6	17–31	e; p; a	M, G, E, F
IL-2	TOGF	4p	0.9	15	e; p; a	T
IL-4	BSF-1	5q	0.9	15–20	e; p; a	T
IL-5	BCGF-II, TRF	5q	1.7	12–18	e; p	T
IL-6	IFN-β2, BSF2	7p21	1.3–1.6	24	p	T, M, F, E, G
IL-7		8q12-13	1.8–2.4	17	a; p	T
IL-9	p40	nr	0.8	40	p	T
Growth factor-inducing factors						
TNF-α	cachectin	6p23	1.6	17	e; p; a	M, T, G, E, F
Lymphotoxin	TNF-β	6p23	1.7	18	e; p	T
IL-6	see above					
IFN-γ	type-II IFN	12	1.7	15–45	p	T
Chemotactic factors						
IL-8	NCF/NAP, TCF	nr	1.8	10	p	M
MCAF		nr	0.7	32	p	M
MIP-1		nr	nr	8–10	p	M
MIP-2		nr	nr	8	p	M
Others						
LIF	HILDA	22q12	4.0	24	p	T, E, F
Activin		nr	nr	nr	e	Sertoli, granulosa cells
Inhibin		nr	nr	32	e	Sertoli, granulosa cells
Oncostatin M		nr	2.0	28	nr	M
TGF-β		nr	1.8	25	p	Plt
Iron-binding proteins		(No cytokines)				
Lactoferin						
Acidic Isoferritin						
Transferrin						

[1] e = Endocrine; p = paracrine; a = autocrine.

[2] T = T lymphocytes; M = monocytes; G = granulocytes; E = endothelial cells; F = fibroblasts; Plt = platelets; SCF = stem cell factor; MGF = mast cell growth factor; T (B) CGF = T (B) cell growth factor; BSF = B-cell-stimulating factor; TGF = transforming growth factor; TRF = T-cell-replacing factor; NCF/NAP = neutrophil chemotactic factor/neutrophil-activating protein; LIF = leukemia inhibitory factor; HILDA = human interleukin for DA cells; MCAF = monocyte chemotactic and activating factor; MIP = macrophage inflammatory protein; nr = not reported.

referred to as multi-CSF) and SCF. IL-3 stimulates the pluripotent stem cell and similar to GM-CSF, immature nonlineage-specific progenitor cells [18, 50, 98, 101]. M-CSF [84, 85], G-CSF [68, 80, 105] and EPO [89, 99] promote maturation of lineage-specific progenitor cells such as colony-forming units (CFU)-G, CFU-M, CFU-MEG or burst-forming units (BFU)-E/CFU-E which will further mature into terminally differentiated cells. In addition, each of these factors also augments the functional capacity of mature end cells. GM-CSF and G-CSF stimulate superoxide production, expression of adhesion molecules and release of lysozyme and elastase by phagocytes [57]. Unlike G-CSF, GM-CSF inhibits migration of neutrophils. Both, GM-CSF and IL-3 enhance cytotoxicity and phagocytosis mediated by eosinophils and stimulate histamine release by basophils [38].

Similar to neutrophils, monocytes express genes of various cytokines and surface-adhesion molecules when exposed to GM-CSF or IL-3, but not G-CSF [39]. M-CSF affects human bone marrow macrophage colony formation only to a limited extent but induces differentiation of monocytes into macrophages and enhances microbicidal and tumoricidal activities of these cells [46, 52, 86, 102, 108]. While other hematopoietic factors fail to stimulate hematopoietic progenitor cells on their own, they may cooperate with CSFs in order to maintain coordinate hematopoiesis. A series of polypeptides which interfere or synergize with CSFs have been identified and the respective genes have been cloned, including IL-1α and IL-1β, IL-2, IL-4, IL-5, IL-6, IL-7, and IL-9. IL-6 and IL-1 support self-renewal and early commitment of pluripotent stem cells in synergy with IL-3 [44, 66, 104]. IL-5 spurs proliferation of the eosinophil lineage [116, 117], while IL-4 synergizes with GM-CSF and EPO to stimulate both granulocyte and erythrocyte formation [79]. IL-4 has also been shown to induce proliferation of connective-tissue-type mast cells and to synergistically support M-CSF cytotoxicity of monocytes [16, 34]. IL-1 and GM-CSF cooperate with M-CSF to stimulate proliferation of macrophage-type colonies [6, 20]. IL-2 is primarily a growth factor for T-cells, but in addition to its suppressive effect on hematopoietic growth via induction of Interferon-gamma (IFNγ), it directly inhibits CSF-mediated proliferation of hematopoietic cells. Under certain conditions, IL-2 may also support the release of GM-CSF and IL-3 by T cells and may thus augment blood cell formation [76].

Another group of hematopoietic growth-promoting cytokines encompass factors which stimulate CSF secretion by bone marrow bystander cells. This group includes TNFα, TNFβ, transforming growth factor-beta (TGFB) [4], leukemia inhibitory factor (LIF) [114], IFNγ [87], IL-1 [36, 37], and IL-6 [59] but also M-CSF, GM-CSF, and IL-3, which, despite their direct growth-promoting effects, also stimulate CSF synthesis by transcriptional or posttranscriptional modifications of CSF gene expression (fig. 3) [42, 55, 62, 77, 111, 113]. TNFα and TNFβ induce cytokine synthesis by monocytes and mesenchymal cells, but synergize with IFNγ in order to directly inhibit growth of hematopoietic cells [14, 24, 26, 49, 74–77]. TGFβ, synthesized by platelets, inhibits proliferation of very early pluripotent stem cells, while more mature progenitor cells appear to be less sensitive to the inhibitory action of this molecule [47].

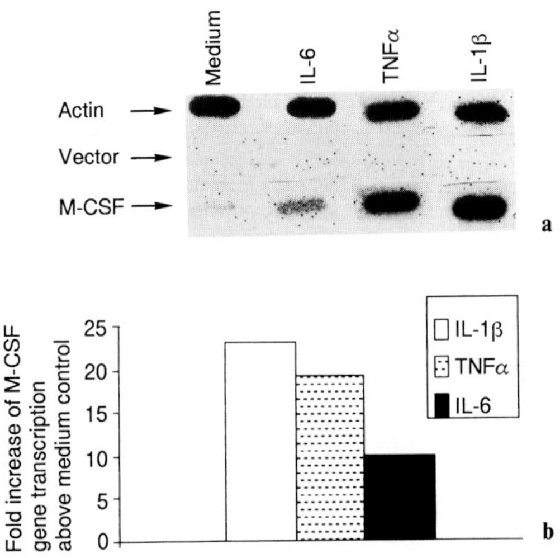

Fig. 3. Enhancement of transcription of the M-CSF gene in monocytes upon in vitro exposure to various cytokines. **a** shows autoradiographs of transcriptional run-on assays performed with monocytes that were treated for 3 h with IL-6, TNFα, or IL-1β. Also transcription of the α-actin gene was analyzed under identical experimental conditions. Plasmids without M-CSF insert (vector) were used as negative controls. **b** Represents a densitometric analysis of the blots shown in **a** to quantitate the fold increase of M-CSF transcription in stimulated cultures above background levels (medium).

Signal Transduction Pathways Involved in Cytokine Gene Activation

Extracellular signals resulting in synthesis of cytokines involve the activation of specific cellular surface receptors. Receptor activation leads to the immediate modulation of cytoplasmic levels of one or more second messengers, which then initiate a cascade of nuclear processes. Main pathways of signal transduction include (1) increase of cyclic AMP and hydrolysis of inositol phospholipids which generate the formation of diacylglycerol and inositol-1,4,5-triphosphate as second messengers; (2) increase in intracellular free calcium concentrations; (3) modulation of the Na^+/H^+ antiport-system that regulate cytosolic pH levels [3, 7, 67, 73]. In this regard, guanine nucleotide binding proteins (G proteins) play a key role, a highly conserved family of proteins that couple receptors to numerous effector systems to activate or inhibit adenylate cyclase, to activate cGMP phosphodiesterase and the phospholipase A_2, C, and D, and that activate protein kinase C (PKC) [21].

Activation of protein kinase C and A results in the phosphorylation of various cellular proteins. Recent studies on the transcriptional regulation of early response genes such as c-fos and c-jun have indicated that artifical perturbations of intracellular second messenger levels can duplicate the physiological effects of growth factors to induce gene expression, thus supporting the notion that second-messenger systems take part in the transcriptional activation of these genes [1].

Signal transduction pathways involved in the regulation of cytokine genes are less well understood. Studies so far reported address primarily the role of PKC activation. We have recently reported that autoinduction of M-CSF by M-CSF in human monocytes involves PKC [12]. A PKC-dependent pathway was also identified in the induction of the IL-2 gene by IL-1 [58]. In addition, phorbolester TPA, a potent activator of PKC, was found to activate IL-1, and TNFα, G-, and GM-CSF [72, 110]. An increase in free cytosolic calcium followed by translocation of PKC is also involved in the activation of the IL-3 gene [33]. Several distinct pathways such as activation of PKC, increase of cAMP or of free cytosolic calcium are reported to mediate the induction of the IL-6 gene [82, 94, 118].

Posttranscriptional Regulation of Cytokine Genes

The posttranscriptional modification of gene transcripts has been shown to represent a poweful tool to control gene expression [13, 14]. To a large extent, the half-life of an mRNA template determines the time for its translation into the corresponding protein. Modification of mRNA stability thus provides an important mechanism to regulate gene expression by bypassing the more complex transcriptional activation. RNAs of regulatory cellular proteins such as proto-oncogenes, growth factors and transcriptional activators are the main targets of posttranscriptional control [32, 81]. Transcripts of these genes tend to have short half-lifes ranging from 10 to 30 min. Structural features (i.e. the AUUUA motive) were identified in the 3'untranslated region of these genes [19] that predispose mRNA to rapid degradation [92, 97]. AU-rich elements have been found in the 3'untranslated region of the G-CSF [19], GM-CSF [92], IL-1, IL-6 and TNFα gene [61], but were not identified in the M-CSF gene [114]. Experimental evidence also suggests that rapidly inducible labile proteins contribute to stabilization or destabilization of certain mRNAs such as c-myc [28] and c-fos [11, 106]. The presence of the protein synthesis inhibitor cycloheximide prolongs the half-life of several cytokine transcripts such as transcripts of GM-CSF [5] and M-CSF [43], suggesting that labile proteins are involved in the destabilization of these transcripts. Various stimuli have been reported to control cytokine gene expression by modification of the transcript half-life (fig. 4). IL-1 causes accumulation of GM-CSF mRNA in vascular endothelial cells by stabilizing the GM-CSF transcript [5]. Addition of the CD 28 antibody to T cells, for example, increases the mRNA half-life of IL-2, IFNγ, GM-CSF and TNFα [56]. Furthermore, the accumulation of M- and GM-CSF transcripts in activated monocytes by endotoxin is exclusively due to delay in mRNA decay and not due to transcriptional activation [30]. Similarly, activation of murine macrophages results in an increase in GM-CSF mRNA mediated by stabilization of the respective transcripts [106]. In addition, both prolongation of the mRNA half-life and reduction of mRNA stability of certain cytokine transcripts were found in myeloid leukemia cells, suggesting that increased mRNA stability may contribute to the pathogenesis of this type of leukemia [30]. Well in line with these data, activation of the N-ras-oncogene by point mutations was found to alter the expression pattern of CSF genes in fibroblasts by increasing the stability of their respective transcripts [27].

Transcriptional Regulation of Cytokine Genes

For most cytokine genes, only small parts of the promoters have been sequenced that extend to up to 500 bp 5′ of the TATA box. High sequence homology between different species such as the mouse and human GM-CSF and IL-4 gene indicates, that the regulation of cytokine genes is conserved during evolution (2, 63, 78, 103]. However, only few regulatory elements common to several cytokine genes have been identified. TNFα, GM-CSF, M-CSF and IL-6 promoter contain binding sites for the NFκB transcription factor [12, 25, 54, 91], a ubiquitous protein which mediates signal transduction between the cytoplasma and the nucleus in many cell types. Binding activity of NFκB can be generated by the tumor promoter TPA and bacterial endotoxin. However, inflammatory lymphokines, such as TNFα, are most potent in this respect [see ref. 53 for review] (fig. 5). Two related, but distinct binding elements, that are recognized by NFκB-like proteins, are termed conserved lymphokine element 1 and 2 (CLE 1 and 2) or cytokine element 1 and 2 (CK1, CK2) [96]. Particularly the CLE1 motive is found in one or more copies in most cytokine genes such as GM-CSF (human and mouse), IL-3, IL-2, G-CSF (human and mouse), IL-4, IL-5 and IL-6, while the CLE2 motive appears to be restricted to the IL-3 and GM-CSF genes [95]. An IL-1 responsive element has recently been described in the IL-6 promoter [45]. IL-1 and IL-6 inducible DNA binding proteins have been described to activate the C-reactive protein [3]. A distinct DNA binding motive appears to be responsible for lymphokine gene activation by the E_2 protein, a bovine papilloma-virus-encoded molecule [35]. Signals leading to T cell activation and the human T cell leukemia virus type I p40x protein activate the GM-CSF gene through the same transcription factor [65]. The transcription factor AP-1, encoded by the c-jun proto-oncogene mediates IL-1 induction of the IL-2 gene [70]. Also TGFβ autoregulates TGFβ expression in fibroblasts via AP-1 [48]. It remains, however, to be seen (1) whether this motive is also present in other cytokine promoters and (2) whether similar specific binding factors can be identified for other lymphokines. The existence of common regulatory elements in the promoter region of various growth factors may contribute to coordinate the induction of some of these genes by a wide range of stimuli.

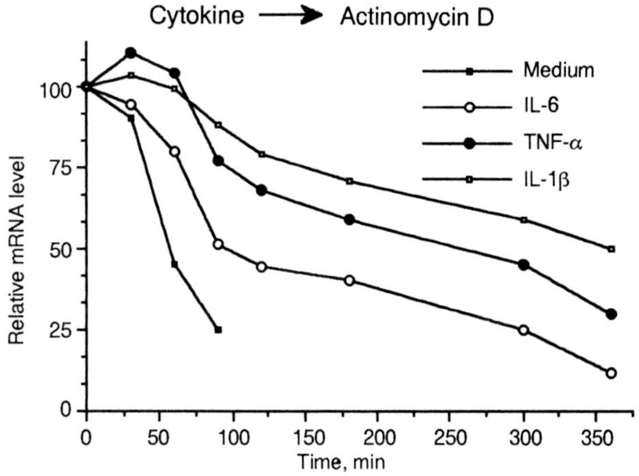

Fig. 4. Effect of treatment of fibroblasts with IL-6 (○), TNFα (●), and IL-1β (□) on decay of M-CSF mRNA. Cells were exposed for 3 h to the inhibitor of gene transcription actinomycin D, given after a 4-hour treatment with or without (medium; ■) IL-6, TNFα, and IL-1β. After the indicated time of culture cytoplasmatic RNA was extracted and hybridized to a M-CSF cDNA. Autoradiographic blots were quantitated by laser densitometry.

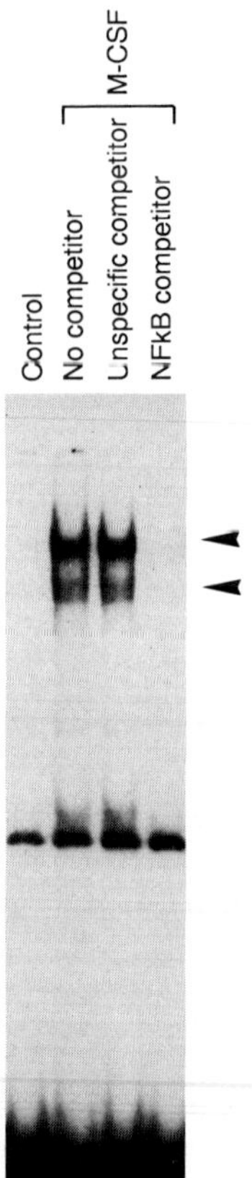

Fig. 5. Autoinduction of M-CSF gene expression by M-CSF in monocytes involves activation of the transcription factor NFκB. A ^{32}P-labeled oligonucleotide containing the HIV-1-κB site was incubated with nuclear extracts obtained from monocytes that were either untreated (control) or treated with M-CSF (no competitor). Nuclear extracts of M-CSF-treated monocytes were incubated with the labeled probe in the presence of 25 n*M* excess of an NFκB-unrelated oligonucleotide (unspecific competitor) or an unlabeled NFκB oligonucleotide (NFκB competitor). The arrows indicate the DNA/NFκB protein binding complex.

References

1 Akashi, M.; Yamoto, K.; Koeffler, H.P.: Hematopoietic growth factors: regulation of production; in Herrmann, Mertelsmann, Hematopoietic growth factors in clinical applications, pp. 41–62 (Dekker, New York 1990).

2 Arai, N.; Nomuura, D.; Villaret, D.; Malefijt, R.D.; Seiki, M.; Yoshida, M.; Minoshima, S.; Fukujama, R.; Maekawa, M.; Kudah, J.: Complete nucleotide sequence of the chromosomal gene for human IL-4 and its expression. J. Immun. *1542:* 247–282 (1989).

3 Aronson, P.; Boron, W.: Na^+/H^+ exchange intracellular pH and cell function, pp. 458–467 (Academic Press, New York 1986).

4 Axelrad, A.A.: Some hematopoietic negative regulators. Exp. Hematol. *18:* 143–150 (1990).

5 Bagby, G.C.; Shaw, G.; Heinrich, M.C.; Hefeneider, S.; Brown, M.A.; De Loughery, T.G.; Segal, G.M.; Band, L.: Interleukin-1 stimulation stabilizes GM-CSF mRNA in human vascular endothelial cells: preliminary studies on the role of the 3'AU-rich motive. Prog. clin. biol. Res. *352:* 233–239 (1990).

6 Bartelmez, S.H.; Stanley, E.R.: Synergism between hematopoietic growth factors (HGFs) detected by their effects on cells bearing receptors for a lineage specific HGF: Assay of hemopoietin. J. cell. Physiol. *122:* 370–378 (1985).

7 Berridge, M.J.; Irvine, R.F.: Inositolphosphates and cell signalling. Nature *431:* 197–205 (1989).

8 Beutler, B.A.; Milsark, I.W.; Cerami, A.: Cachectin/tumor necrosis factor: production, distribution, and metabolic fate in vivo. J. Immun. *135:* 3972–3977 (1985).

9 Bond, M.W.; Schrader, B.; Mosmann, T.R.; Coffmann, R.L.: A mouse T-cells: product that preferentially enhances IgA production. II. Physiochemical characterization. J. Immun. *138:* 3691–3696 (1987).

10 Brach, M.A.; Cicco, N.A.; Riedel, D.; Hirano, T.; Kishimoto, T.; Mertelsmann, R.H.; Herrmann, F.: Mechanism of differential regulation of IL-6 mRNA accumulation by tumor necrosis factor alpha and lymphotoxin during monocytic differentiation. FEBS Lett. *263:* 349–354 (1990).

11 Brach, M.A.; Henschler, R.; Mertelsmann, R.; Herrmann, F.: Regulation of M-CSF expression by M-CSF: role of proteinkinase C and transcription factor NFkappa B. Pathobiol. *59:* 284–288 (1991).

12 Brach, M.A.; Riedel, D.; Mertelsmann, R.; Herrmann, F.: Induction of monocytic differentiation and modulation of expression of proto-oncogenes in human leukemic monoblasts by cytokines and phorbolester. Virchows Arch. [B] *59:* 54–59 (1990).

13 Brawerman, C.: Determinants of messenger RNA stability. Cell *48:* 5–6 (1987).

14 Brawerman, G.: mRNA decay finding the right targets. Cell *57:* 9–10 (1989).

15 Broudy, V.C.; Kaushansky, K.; Segal, G.M.; Harlan, J.M.; Adamson, J.W.: Tumor necrosis factor alpha stimulates human endothelial cells to produce granulocyte-macrophage colony stimulating factor. Proc. natn. Acad. Sci. USA *83:* 7467–7471 (1986).

16 Brown, M.A.; Pierce, J.H.; Watson, C.J.; Falco, I.; Ihle, J.N.; Paul, W.E.: B-cell stimulatory factor/interleukin-4 mRNA is expressed by normal and transformed mast cells. Cell *50:* 804–818 (1987).

17 Broxmeyer, H.E.: Biomolecule-interactions and the regulation of myelopoiesis. Int. J. Cell Cloning *4:* 378–404 (1986).

18 Burgess, A.W.; Bergley, C.G. Johnson, G.R.; Lopez, A.F.; Wiliamson, D.J.; Mermod, J.J.; Simpson, R.J.; Schmitz, A.; de Lamarter, J.F.: Purification and properties of bacterial synthesized human granulocyte-macrophage colony stimulating factor. Blood *69:* 43–51 (1987).

19 Caput, D.; Beutler, B.; Hartog, K.; Thayer, R.; Brown-Shimer, S.; Cerami, A.: Identification of a common nucleotide sequence in the 3'untranslated region of mRNA molecules specifying inflammatory mediators. Proc. natn. Acad. Sci. USA *83:* 1670–1674 (1986).

20 Caracciolo, D.; Shisat, N.; Wong, G.; Lange, B.; Clark, S.; Rovera, G.: Recombinant human macrophage-colony stimulating factor (M-CSF) requires subliminal concentrations of granulocyte-macrophage (GM-)CSF for optimal stimulation of human macrophage colony stimulation in vitro. J. exp. Med. *166:* 1851–1860 (1987).

21 Casey, P.J.; Gelman, A.G.: G proteins: Involvement on receptor effector coupling. J. Biol. Chem. *263:* 2577–2586 (1988).

22 Cline, M.J.; Golde, D.W.: Cellular interactions in hematopoiesis. Nature *277:* 177–181 (1979).

23 Coffman, R.L.; Schrader, B.; Casty, J.; Mosmann, T.R.; Bond, M.W.: A mouse T-cell product that preferentially enhances IgA production. I. Biological characterization. J. Immun. *138:* 3685–3690 (1987).

24 Collart, M.A.; Belin, D.; Vassali, J.D.; Kowodo, S.; Vassali, P.: Gamma-Interferon enhances macrophage-transcription of the tumor necrosis factor/cachetin, interleukin-1 and urokinase gene which are controlled by short-lived repressors. J. exp. Med. *164:* 2113–2118 (1986).

25 Collart, M.A.; Baeuerle, P.; Vassali, P.: Regulation of tumor necrosis factor alpha transcription in macrophages: Involvement of four kB like motifs and of constitutive and inducible forms of NFkB. Mol. cell. Biol. *10:* 1498–1506 (1990).

26 V. Damme, J.; Opdenakker, G.; Simpson, R.J.; Rubira, M.R.; Cauphas, S.; Vink, A.; Billiau, A.; van Snick, J.: Identification of the human 26-kD protein, interferon beta as a B cell hybridoma/plasmocytoma growth factor induced by interleukin-1 and tumor necrosis factor. J. exp. Med. *165.* 914–919 (1987).

27 Demetri, G.D.; Ernst, T.J.; Zenzi, B.W.: Transfection of the EJ-ras oncogene into fibroblasts alters expression of genes for colony stimulating factors and interleukin-1. Blood *72:* suppl. 1, 113 (1988).

28 Dony, C.; Kessel, M.; Gruss, P.: Posttranscriptional control of myc and p53 expression during differentiation of the embryonal carcinoma cell line F9. Nature *317:* 636–639 (1988).

29 Dutton, R.; Hoffmann, M.: Immune response restoration with macrophage culture supernatants. Science *172:* 1047–1048 (1971).

30 Ernst, T.J.; Ritchie, A.R.; Demetri, G.D.; Griffin, J.D.: Regulation of granulocyte and macrophage stimulating factor mRNA levels in human blood monocytes is mediated primarily at a posttranscriptional level. J. biol. Chem. *264:* 5700–5706 (1989).

31 Ganter, U.; Arcone, R.; Toniatti, C.; Morrone, G.; Ciliberto, G.: Dual control of C-reactive protein gene expression by interleukin-1 and interleukin 6. EMBO J. *8:* 3773–3779 (1989).

32 Greenberg, M.E.; Hermanowski, A.L.; Ziff, E.B.: Effect of protein synthesis inhibitors on growth factor activation of c-fos,

c-myc, and actin gene transcription. Mol. cell. Biol. *6:* 1050–1056 (1986).

33 Gelfland, E.; Cheung, R.K.; Grunstein, S.: Calcium-dependent intracellular acidification dominates the pH response to mitogen in human T-cells. J. Immun. *144:* 246–252 (1988).

34 Hamaguchi, Y.; Kanakura, Y.; Fujita, J.; Takeda, S.I.; Nakano, T.; Tarui, S.; Honjo, T.; Kitamura, Y.: Interleukin 4 as an essential factor for in vitro growth of murine connective tissue-type mast cells. J. exp. Med. *165:* 268–273 (1987).

35 Heike, T.; Miyatake, S.; Yoshida, M., Arai, K.; Arai, N.: Bovine papilloma virus encoded E2 protein activates lymphokine genes through DNA elements distinct from the consensus motive in the control region of its own genome. EMBO J. *8:* 1411–1417 (1989).

36 Herrmann, F.; Oster, W.; Meuer, S.C.; Lindemann, A.; Mertelsmann, R.: Interleukin-1 induces T cell production of granulocyte-macrophage colony stimulating factor. J. clin. Invest. *81:* 1415–1418 (1988).

37 Herrmann, F.; Cannistra, S.A.; Lindemann, A.; Rambaldi, A.; Mertelsmann, R.; Griffin, J.D.: Functional consequences of monocyte-interleukin-2-receptor expression: Induction of interleukin-1 secretion by gamma interferon and interleukin-2. J. Immun. *142:* 139–145 (1989).

38 Herrmann, F.; Mertelsmann, R.: Polypeptides controlling hematopoietic cell development and activation. I. In vitro results. Blut *58:* 117–128 (1989).

39 Herrmann, F.: Neutropenia and its treatment with recombinant hematopoietic growth factors. Clinician *8:* 2–11 (1990).

40 Herrmann, F.; Mertelsmann, R.: Regulatory effects of cytokines on myelopoiesis; in Coffey (ed.), Granulocyte response to hematopoietic growth factors (Dekker, New York, in press).

41 Hirano, T.; Yasukawa, K.; Harada, H.; Taga, T.; Watanabe, Y.; Matsuda, T.; Kashiwamura, S.; Nakajuma, K.; Koyama, K.; Iwamatsu, A.; Trunasawa, S.; Sakiyama, F.; Matusi, H.; Takahara, Y.; Taniguchi, T.; Kishimoto, T.: Complementary DNA for a novel human interleukin (BSF-2) that induces B-lymphocytes to produce immunoglobulin. Nature *324:* 73–76 (1986).

42 Horiguchi, J.; Warren, K.M.; Kufe, D.: Expression of the macrophage-specific colony stimulating factor in human monocytes treated with granulocyte-macrophage colony stimulating factor. Blood *69:* 1259–1261 (1987).

43 Horiguchi, J.; Sariban, E.; Kufe, D.: Transcriptional and post-transcriptional regulation of CSF-1 gene expression in human monocytes. Mol. cell. Biol. *8:* 3951–3954 (1988).

44 Ikebuchi, K.; Wong, G.G.; Clark, S.C.; Ihle, J.N.; Ogawa, M.: Interleukin-6 enhancement of IL-3 dependent proliferation of multipotential hematopoietic precursors. Proc natn. Acad Sci. USA *84:* 9035–9039 (1987).

45 Isshiki, H.; Akira, S.; Tanabe, O.; Nakajima, T.; Shimamoto, T.; Hirano, T.; Kishimoto, T.: Constitutive and interleukin-1 (IL-1) inducible factors interact with the IL-1 responsive element in the IL-6 gene. Mol. cell. Biol. *10:* 2757–2764 (1990).

46 Karbassi, A.; Becker, J.M.; Foster, J.S.; Moore, R.N.: Enhanced killing of *Candida albicans* by murine macrophages treated with macrophage-colony stimulating factor: evidence for augmented expression of mannose receptors. J. Immun. *139:* 417–423 (1987).

47 Keller, J.R.; Mantel, C.; Sing, G.K.; Ellingworth, C.R.; Ruscetti, S.K.; Ruscetti, F.W.: Transforming growth factor-beta-1 selectively regulates early murine hematopoietic progenitors and inhibits the growth of IL-3 dependent myeloid leukemia cell lines. J. exp. Med. *168:* 737–742 (1988).

48 Kirn, S.J.; Angel, P.; Lafyatis, R.; Hattori, K.; Kim, K.Y.; Sporn, M.B.; Karin, M.; Roberts, A.B.: Autoinduction of transforming growth factor beta is mediated by the AP-1 complex. Mol. cell. Biol. *10:* 1492–1497 (1990).

49 Koeffler, H.P.; Gasson, J.; Ranyard, J.; Souza, L.; Shepard, M.; Munker, R.: Recombinant humann TNF-alpha stimulates production of granulocyte-colony stimulating factor. Blood *70:* 55–59 (1987).

50 Leary, A.G.; Yang, Y.C.; Clark, S.C.; Gasson, J.C.; Golde, D.W.; Ogawa, M.: Recombinant gibbon Interleukin-3 supports formation of human multilineage colonies and blast cell colonies in culture: comparison with recombinant human granulocyte-macrophage colony-stimulating factor. Blood *70:* 1343–1348 (1987).

51 Lee, M.T.; Warren, M.K.: CSF-1 induced resistance to viral infection in murine macrophages. J. Immun. *139:* 3019–3024 (1987).

52 Lee, F.; Yokota, T.; Otsuka, T.; Meyerson, P.; Villaret, D.; Coffman, R.; Mosmann, T.; Rennick, D.; Roehm, N.; Smith, C.: Isolation and charcterization of a mouse interleukin-cDNA clone that express B-cell stimulatory factor-1 activities and T-cell and mast-cell activities. Proc. natn. Acad. Sci. USA *83:* 2061–2065 (1986).

53 Leonardo, M.J.; Baltimore, D.: NFκB: a pleiotropic mediator of inducible and tissue-specific gene control. Cell *58:* 227–229 (1989).

54 Liberman, T.A.; Baltimore, D.: Activation of interleukin-6 gene expression through the NFκB transcription factor. Mol. cell. Biol. *10:* 2327–2334 (1990).

55 Lindemann, A.; Oster, W.; Ziegler-Heitbrock, H.W.L.; Mertelsmann, R.; Herrmann, F.: Recombinant granulocyte-macrophage colony stimulating factor induces monokine secretion by polymorphonuclear leukocytes. J. clin. Invest. *898:* 1308–1314 (1989).

56 Lindsten, T.; June, C.H.; Ledbetter, J.A.; Stella, G.; Thompson, C.B.: Regulation of lymphokine messenger RNA stability by a surface-mediated T-cell activation pathway. Science *244:* 339–343 (1989).

57 Lübbert, M.; Herrmann, F.; Koeffler, H.P.: Expression and regulation of myeloid-specific genes in normal and leukemic myeloid cells. Blood *77:* 909–924 (1991).

58 Macchia, G.; Baldari, C.T.; Massone, A.; Tilford, I.L.: A role of protein kinase C activity in interleukin-I (IL-1) induction of the IL-2 gene expression but not in IL 1 signal transduction. Mol. cell. Biol. *10:* 2731–2737 (1990).

59 Mantovani, L.; Henschler, R.; Brach, M.A.; Wieser, R.; Lübbert, M.; Lindemann, A.; Mertelsmann, R.H.; Herrmann, F.: Differential regulation of interleukin-6 expression in human fibroblasts by tumor necrosis factor-a and lymphotoxin. FEBS Lett. *270:* 152–156 (1990).

60 Mantovani, L.; Henschler, R.; Brach, M.A.; Mertelsmann, R.; Herrmann, F.: Regulation of gene-expression of M-CSF by acute phase response proteins in human fibroblasts. FEBS Lett. *280:* 97–102 (1991).

61 Matsuda, T.; Suematsu, S.; Kawano, M.; Yoshizaki, K.; Akira, S.; Hirano, T.; Kishimoto, T.: IL-6/BSF2 in normal and abnormal regulation of immune responses; in Sehgal, Grienin-

ger, Tosato, Regulation of the acute phase and immune responses: IL-6. Ann. N.Y. Acad. Sci. *557:* 466–477 (1989).
62 Metcalf, D.; Nicola, N.A.: Synthesis by mouse peritoneal cells of G-CSF, the differentiation inducer for myeloid leukemia cells: stimulation by endotoxin, MCSF and multi-CSF. Leuk. Res. *9:* 35–50 (1985).
63 Miyatake, S.; Otsuka, T.; Yokota, T.; Lee, F.; Arai, K.: Structure of the chromosomal gene for granulocyte-macrophage colony stimulating factor: comparison of the mouse and human genes. EMBO J. *4:* 2561–2568 (1985).
64 Miyatake, S.; Seiki, M.; Malefit, R.D.; Heike, T.; Fusijawa, J.; Takebe, Y.; Nishida, J.; Shlomat, J.; Yokota, T.; Yoshida, M.: Activation of T-cell derived lymphokine genes in T-cells and fibroblasts. Effect of human T-cell leukemia virus type p40x protein and bovine papilloma virus encoded E2 protein. Nucleic Acids Res. *14:* 6547–6566 (1988).
65 Miyatake, S.; Seiki, M.; Yoshida, M.; Arai, K.: T-cell activation signals and human T-cell leukemia virus type I-encoded p40x protein activate the mouse granulocyte-macrophage colony-stimulating factor gene through a common DNA element. Mol. cell. Biol. *8:* 5581–5587 (1988).
66 Mochizuki, D.Y.; Eisenmann, J.R.; Conlon, P.J.; Larsen, A.D.; Tushinski, R.J.: Interleukin 1 regulates hematopoietin activity, a role previously ascribed to hematopoietin 1. Proc. natn. Acad. Sci. USA *84:* 5267–5271 (1987).
67 Moolenar, W.H.: Ionic signals in the activation of growth factors. Ann N.Y. Acad. Sci. *551:* 179–184 (1988).
68 Moore, M.A.S.; Welte, K.; Gabrilove, J.; Souza, L.M.: Biological activities of recombinant human granulocyte colony stimulating factor (rh G-CSF) and tumor necrosis factor: in vivo and in vitro analysis. Haematol. Blood Transfus. *31:* 210–220 (1987).
69 Morgan, D.A.; Ruscetti, F.W.; Gallo, R.: Selctive in vitro growth of T-lymphocyte from normal human bone marrow. Science *193:* 1007–1008 (1976).
70 Muegge, K.; Williams, T.M.; Kant, J.; Marin, M.; Chiu, R.; Schmidt, A.; Siebenlist, U.; Young, H.A.; Durum, S.K.: Interleukin-1 constimulatory activity on the interleukin-2 promotor via AP-1. Science *246:* 249–251 (1989).
71 Munker, R.; Gasson, J.; Ogawa, M.; Koeffler, H.P.: Recombinant human TNF induces production of granulocyte monocyte colony stimulating factor. Nature *323:* 79–82 (1986).
72 Nimer, S.D.; Gates, M.J.; Koeffler, H.P.; Gasson, J.C.: Multiple mechanism control the expression of granulocyte-macrophage colony-stimulating factor by human fibroblasts. J. Immun. *143:* 2374–2377 (1989).
73 Nishizuka, Y.: The molecular heterogeneity of protein kinase C and its implication for cellular regulation. Nature *334:* 661–665 (1988).
74 Oster, W.; Lindemann, A.; Mertelsmann, R.; Herrmann, F.: GM-CSF and multi-CSF regulate monocyte secretion of G-CSF. Blood *73:* 64–70 (1989).
75 Oster, W.; Lindemann, A.; Horn, S.; Mertelsmann, R.; Herrmann, F.: Tumor necrosis factor (TNF) alpha but not TNF-beta induces secretion of colony stimulating factor for macrophages by human monocytes. Blood *70:* 1700–1703 (1987).
76 Oster, W.; Lindemann, A.; Horn, S.; Mertelsmann, R.; Herrmann, F.: Gene expression and production of M-, G-, GM-CSF, and multi-CSF in the peripheral blood. Eur. J. Immun. *19:* 453–459 (1989).
77 Oster, W.; Lindemann, A.; Mertelsmann, R.; Herrmann F.: Gamma interferon regulates secretion of G-CSF in human monocytes at the transcriptional level; in Camntrell, Schellekens, The biology of the interferon system, pp. 243–250 (Nijhoff, Dordrecht 1987).
78 Otsuka, T.; Villaret, D.; Yokota, T.; Takebe, Y.; Lee, F.: Structural analysis of the mouse chromosomal gene encoding interleukin-4 which expresses B-cell, T-cell and mast-cell stimulatory activities. Nucleic Acids Res. *15:* 333–344 (1987).
79 Peschel, C.; Paul, W.; Ohara, J.; Green, I.: Effect of B cell stimulatory factor-1/interleukin 4 on hematopoietic progenitor cells. Blood *70:* 254–263 (1987).
80 Platzer, E.; Welte, K.; Gabrilove, J.L.; Lu, L.; Harris, P.; Mertelsmann, R.; Moore, M.A.S.: Biological activities of human pluripotent hemopoietic colony stimulating factor on normal and leukemic cells. J. exp. Med. *162:* 1788–1801 (1985).
81 Raj, N.B.K.; Pitha, P.M.: Two levels of beta interferon gene expression in human cells. Proc. natn. Acad. Sci. USA *80:* 3923–3927 (1983).
82 Ray, A.; Tatter, S.B.; May, L.T.; Seghal, P.B.: Activation of the human beta interferon/hepatocyte-stimulatory factor/interleukin-6 promotor by cytokines, viruses and second messenger agonists. Proc. natn. Acad. Sci. USA *85:* 6701–6705 (1988).
83 Ray, A.; Tatter, S.B.; Santhanam, U.; Helfgott, D.C.; May, L.T.; Sehgal, P.: Regulation of expression of interleukin-6. Molecular and clinical studies; in Sehgal, Grieninger, Tosato, Regulation of the acute phase and immune response. Ann. N.Y. Acad. Sci. *557:* 353–361 (1989).
84 Ralph, P.; Warren, M.K.; Nakoinz, I.; Lee, M.T.; Brindley, L.; Samspon-Johannes, A.; Kawasaki, E.S.; Ladner, M.B.; Strickler, J.E.; Boosman, A.; Csejetey, J.; White, T.: Biological properties and molecular biology of the human macrophage growth factor CSF-1. Immunobiology *172:* 194–204 (1986).
85 Ralph, P.: Molecular properties and biological activity of human macrophage colony stimulating growth factor CSF-1. Haematol. Blood Transfus. *31:* 221–227 (1987).
86 Ralph, P.; Nakoinz, J.: Stimulation of macrophage tumoricidal activity by the growth and differentiation factor CSF-1. Cell. Immunol. *105:* 270–279 (1987).
87 Reem, G.H.; Yeh, N.H.: Interleukin 2 regulates the expression of its receptor and synthesis of gamma interferon by human T-lymphocytes. Science *225:* 429–431 (1984).
88 Rysek, R.P.; Hirai, S.I.; Yaniv, M.; Bravo, R.: Transcriptional activation of c-jun during the Go/Go1 transition in mouse fibroblasts. Nature *334:* 535–537 (1988).
89 Sakaguchi, M.; Kawakita, M.; Matsuhita, H.J.; Shibuja K.; Koishihara, Y.; Takatsuki, K.: Human erythropoietin stimulates murine megakaryopoiesis in serum-free culture. Exp. Hematol. *15:* 1028–1034 (1987).
90 Schimpf, A.; Wecker, E.: Replacement of T-cell function by a T-cell product. Nature *237:* 15–17 (1972).
91 Schreck, R.; Baeuerle, P.: NFκB as inducible transcriptional activator of the granulocyte-macrophage colony stimulating factor gene. Mol. cell. Biol. *10:* 1281–1286 (1990).
92 Schuler, G.D.; Cole, M.D.: GM-CSF and oncogene mRNA stabilities are independently regulated in trans in a mouse monocytic tumor. Cell *55:* 1115–1122 (1988).
93 Seelentag, W.K.; Mermod, J.J.; Montenaso, R.; Vassalli, P.: Additive effects of interleukin-1 and tumor necrosis factor on the accumulation of three granulocyte and macrophage colony

stimulating factor mRNAs in human endothelial cells. EMBO J. *6:* 2261–2265 (1987).
94 Sehgal, P.B.; Walther, Z.; Tamm, I.: Rapid enhancement of beta-2 interferon/B-cell differentiation factor BSF-2 gene expression in human fibroblasts by diacylglycerol and the calcium ionophore A 23187. Proc. natn. Acad. Sci. USA *84:* 3663–3667 (1987).
95 Shannon, M.F.; Pell, L.M.; Leonardo, M.J.; Kuczek, E.S.; Occhiodoro, F.S.; Dunn, S.M.; Vadas, M.A.: A novel tumor necrosis factor-responsive transcription factor which recognizes a regulatory element in hemopoietic growth factor genes. Mol. cell. Biol. *10:* 2950–2959 (1990).
96 Shannon, M.F.; Gamble, J.R.; Vadas, M.A.: Nuclear proteins interacting with the promotor region of the human granulocyte/macrophage colony stimulating factor gene. Proc. natn. Acad. Sci. USA *85:* 674–678 (1988).
97 Shaw, G.; Kamen, R.: A conserved AU sequence from the 3'untranslated region of the GM-CSF mRNA mediates selective mRNA degradation. Cell *46:* 659–665 (1986).
98 Sieff, C.A.; Emerson, S.G.; Donahue, R.E.; Nathan, D.G.; Wang, E.A.; Wong, C.G.; Clark, S.C.: Human recombinant granulocyte-macrophage colony stimulating factor: a multilineage hematopoietin. Science *230:* 1171–1173 (1985).
99 Sieff, C.A.; Niemeyer, C.M.; Nathan, D.G.; Ekem, S.C.; Bieber, F.R.; Yang, Y.C.; Wong, G.; Clark, S.C.: Stimulation of human hematopoietic colony formation be recombinant gibbon multi-colony stimulating factor or interleukin-3. J. clin. Invest. *80:* 818–823 (1987).
100 Sieff, C.A.; Emerson, S.G.; Mufson, A.; Gesner, T.G.; Nathan, D.G.: Dependence of highly enriched bone marrow progenitors on hemopoietic growth factors and their response to recombinant erythropoietin. J. clin. Invest. *77:* 74–81 (1986).
101 Sieff, C.A.; Schickwann, T.; Taller, V.: Interleukin 1 induces cultured human endothelial cell production of granulocyte-macrophage colony-stimulating factor. J. clin. Invest. *79:* 48–51 (1987).
102 Stanley, E.R.; Guilberte, L.J.; Tushinski, R.R.; Bartelmez, S.H.: CSF-1 a mononuclear phagocyte lineage specific hemopoietic growth factor. J. cell. Biochem. *21:* 151–156 (1983).
103 Stanley, E.; Metcalf, D.; Sobieszczuk, P.; Gough, N.M.; Dunn, A.R.: The structure and expression of the murine gene encoding granulocyte-macrophage colony-stimulating factor: Evidence for utilization of alternative promotors. EMBO J. *4:* 2569–2573 (1985).
104 Stanley, E.R.; Bartocci, A.; Patinkin, D.; Rosendaal, M.; Bradley, T.R.: Regulation of very primitive, multipotent hemopoietic cells by hemopoietin-1. Cell *45:* 667–674 (1986).
105 Souza, L.M.; Boone, T.C.; Gabrilove, J.L.; Lai, P.H.; Zsebo, K.M.; Murdock, D.C.; Chazin, V.R.; Bruszewski, J.; Lu, H.; Chen, K.K.; Barendt, J.; Platzer, E.; Moore, M.A.S.; Mertelsmann, R.; Welte, K.: Recombinant human granulocyte colony stimulating factor: effects on normal and leukemic myeloid cells. Science *232:* 61–65 (1987).
106 Thorens, B.; Mermod, J.J.; Vassalli, P.: Phagocytosis and inflammatory stimuli induce GM-CSF mRNA in macrophages through posttranscriptional regulation. Cell *48:* 671–678 (1987).
107 Treismann, R.: Transient accumulation of c-fos RNA following serum stimulation requires a conserved 5'element and c-fos 3'sequences. Cell *42:* 889–902 (1985).
108 Tushinski, R.J.; Stanley, E.R.: The regulation of macrophage protein turnover by a colony stimulating factor CSF-1. J. cell. Physiol. *116:* 67–73 (1983).
109 Unanue, E.R.: Cooperation between mononuclear phagocytes and lymphocytes in immunity. New Engl. J. Med. *303:* 977–892 (1980).
110 Updyke, L.W.; Yoom, H.L.; Chuthaputti, H.; Pfeiffer, R.W.; Yim, G.K.: Induction of interleukin-1 and tumor necrosis factor by TPA in phorbol ester-sensitive (SENCAR) and resistant (B6C3FI) mice. Carcinogenesis *10:* 1107–1111 (1989).
111 Vellenga, E.; Rambaldi, A.; Ernst, T.; Ostapovicz, D.; Griffin, J.D. The G-CSF and GM-CSF genes are independently regulated in human monocytes. Blood *70:* 1529–1532 (1988).
112 Witte, O.N.: Steel locus defines new multipotent growth factor. Cell *63:* 5–6 (1990).
113 Warren, M.K.; Ralph, P.: Macrophage growth factor (CSF-1) stimulates human monocyte production of interferon, tumor necrosis factor and colony stimulating activity. J. Immun. *137:* 2281–2285 (1986).
114 Williams, R.L.; Hilton, D.J.; Pease, S.; Willson, T.A.; Stewart, C.L.; Gearing, D.P.; Wagner, E.F.; Metcalf, D.; Nicola, N.A.; Gough, N.M.: Myeloid leukaemia inhibitory factor maintains the developmental potential of embryonic stem cells. Nature *336:* 684–686 (1988).
115 Wong, G.G.; Temple, P.A.; Leary, A.C.; Witek-Gianotti, J.A.; Yang, Y.; Ciarletta, A.; Chun, M.; Murtha, P.; Kriz, R.; Kaufman, R.J.; Ferenz, C.R.; Sibley, B.S.; Turner, K.; Hewick, R.; Clark, S.C.; Amadi, N.; Yokota, H.; Yamada, M.; Saito, M.; Motoyoshi, K.; Fuminaro, T.: Human CSF-1: molecular cloning and expression of a 4kB cDNA encoding the human urinary protein. Science *235:* 1504–1509 (1987).
116 Yang, Y.C.; Ciarletta, A.B.; Temple, P.A.; Chung, M.P.; Kovacic, S.; Witek-Geanotti, J.S.; Leary, A.C.; Kriz, R.; Donahue, R.E.; Wong, G.G.; Clark S.C.: Human IL-3 (multi-CSF): Identification by expression cloning of a novel hematopoietic growth factor related to murine IL-3. Cell *47:* 3–10 (1986).
117 Yokota T.; Coffman, R.L.; Hagiwara, H.; Rennick, D.M.; Takebe, Y; Yokota, K.; Gemmel, L.; Shrader, B.; Yang, G.; Meyerson, P.; Luh, J.; Hoy, P.; Pene, J.; Briere, F.; Spits, H.; Bachereau, J.; de Vries, J.; Lee, F.D.; Arai, N.; Arai, K.I.: Isolation and characterization of lymphokine cDNA clones encoding mouse and human IgA-enhancing factor and eosinophil colony-stimulating activities; Relationship to interleukin 5. Proc. natn. Acad. Sci. USA *84:* 7388–7392 (1987).
118 C Zhang, YH.; Lin, J.; Vilcek, J.: Enhancement of cAMP levels and of protein kinase activity by tumor necrosis factor and interleukin-1 in human fibroblasts: role in the induction of interleukin-6. Proc. natn. Acad. Sci. USA *85:* 6802–6805 (1988).

Prof. Dr. F. Herrmann
Department of Hematology and Oncology
University of Freiburg Medical Center
Hugstetter Str. 55
D-W-7800 Freiburg (FRG)

Acta Haematol 1991;86:138–147

0001–5792/91/0863–0138 $2.75/0

Clinical Role of Colony Stimulating Factors

W. Brugger, F.M. Rosenthal, L. Kanz, R. Mertelsmann

Department of Hematology and Oncology, University Medical Center, Freiburg, FRG

Key Words. Cytokines · Erythropoietin · Hematology · Hematopoietic growth factors · Oncology

Introduction

Hematopoiesis is sustained throughout life by a small pool of pluripotent hematopoietic stem cells, which have the capacity for both self-renewal and multilineage differentiation into myeloid, erythroid, megakaryocytic and lymphoid lineages. Stem cells give rise to lineage-restricted progenitor cells that in turn proliferate and differentiate into mature blood cells. The proliferation and differentiation of progenitor cells in vivo is controlled by a network of stimulatory and inhibitory hormones and by interactions with bone marrow stromal cells. Within the stimulatory hormones, colony-simulating factors (CSF) or hematopoietic growth factors are most important.

Since progenitor cells can be identified in vitro only by their ability to form colonies upon stimulation with specific CSFs, the development of semisolid colony-forming assays [1, 2] provided the possibility to distinguish and purify them from conditioned media and from human urine. These colony-stimulating factors include glycoproteins which directly stimulate colony formation of myeloid progenitor cells and/or erythroid progenitors in vitro: granulocyte-macrophage colony-stimulating factor (GM-CSF), granulocyte colony-stimulating factor (G-CSF), macrophage colony-stimulating factor (M-CSF), multi-colony-stimulating factor or interleukin-3 (multi-CSF or IL-3), IL-5 and erythropoietin (EPO). In addition, several other hematopoietic growth factors (IL-1, IL-4, IL-6 IL-7, IL-11 and stem cell factor) have been identified and were shown to have actions on myeloid and lymphoid stem and progenitor cells.

During the past 6 years, the genes, chromosomal localizations and most receptor molecules have been identified and the recombinant proteins of these growth factors revolutionized experimental and clinical hematology. The availability of large amounts of purified recombinant CSF made it possible to initiate clinical trials, and today they open new opportunities for the treatment of a variety of neoplastic disorders. This article will briefly review some of the possible clinical applications of CSF (table 1) and discuss future prospects.

Correction of Insufficient Hematopoiesis

Treatment of Anemia with EPO

EPO is the principal factor controlling red cell production [3]. It acts on erythroid progenitor cells in the bone marrow (CFU-E, BFU-E) [4] and is produced primarily by peritubular interstitial cells of the kidney [5, 6]. Its synthesis is stimulated by decreased oxygen delivery; the oxygen sensor is a heme protein. Extrarenal production occurs in the liver and in bone marrow macrophages [7, 8]. It was originally purified from urine of patients with aplastic anemia [9] and identified as an acidic glycoprotein consisting of 166 amino acids with a molecular weight of 34 kD; its gene is located on chromosome 7q [10]. The murine EPO receptor gene has been cloned [11] and more recently, the coding sequence of the human EPO receptor has been analysed and assigned to chromosome 19p [12, 13]. This receptor belongs to a new receptor family (= cytokine receptor family) which comprises the IL-2 receptor β-subunit and the receptors for IL-3, IL-4, IL-5, IL-6, IL-7, G-CSF and GM-CSF [14–18].

Treatment of anemia with recombinant human EPO was initially done in patients with end-stage renal disease, a disorder characterized by reduced EPO serum levels. Clinical studies have demonstrated its efficacy in these patients [19, 20] as well as in predialysis patients [21, 22]. Those patients received 50–300 units per kilogram of body weight (three times weekly) either intravenously or subcutaneously. After 12 weeks of treatment, nearly all study patients showed a marked increase in reticulocytes, hemoglobin and hematocrit with complete disappearance of any transfusion requirement.

In additional studies it was documented that EPO may be effective in patients with severe anemia with normal renal function, e.g. in the treatment of anemia associated with multiple myeloma [23], neoplastic bone marrow infiltration [24], in AIDS patients treated with zidovudine (AZT) [25], in chronic rheumatoid arthritis [26], in correcting chemotherapy-induced anemia [27, 28] or anemia associated with cancer [29]. These patients were shown to have an inappropriately low EPO serum level as compared to patients with a comparable degree of anemia caused by iron deficiency [30]. However, in patients with dyserythropoiesis (e.g. myelodysplastic syndromes), EPO therapy was beneficial only in a very small number of patients [own results, manuscript in preparation]. Another possible application of EPO is the increased preoperative collection of autologous blood before elective surgery [31].

No major side effects were seen during EPO therapy in patients with normal renal function. In patients with end-stage renal disease, however, EPO therapy was sometimes associated with hypertension, strokes, seizures and increased blood viscosity. In patients with preexisting iron overload, iron stores were decreased by EPO therapy.

Acceleration of Hematological Recovery following Chemotherapy ± Autologous Bone Marrow Transplantation

Delayed hemopoietic recovery following intensive chemotherapy with or without autologous bone marrow support represents one of the major problems in clinical oncology.

Despite considerable improvements in supportive care, bacterial and fungal infections and bleeding complications remain the major risks during the pancytopenic period following intensive chemotherapy.

Therefore, based on their ability to stimulate progenitor cell proliferation and differentiation as well as the functional activity of mature blood cells, the CSFs may be used to reduce morbidity induced by intensive anticancer treatment, to avoid delays between chemotherapy cycles and to allow investigation of dose intensification in selected patient groups.

Table 1. Potential applications of CSFs

Correction of insufficient hematopoiesis:
Treatment of Anemia
Prevention of chemotherapy-induced neutropenia
Possibility of dose intensification
Autologous bone marrow transplantation
Stimulation of hematopoiesis in primary bone marrow failure
Aplastic anemia
Congenital neutropenia or other idiopathic cytopenias
Use in the treatment of leukemias
Treatment of acute myeloid leukemia
Myelodysplastic syndromes
Expansion and recruitment of circulating progenitor cells
Peripheral blood stem cell transplantation
Activation of effector cell function
Infections
Leukocyte function disorders
AIDS
Tumor cytotoxicity

Currently, IL-3, GM-CSF, G-CSF and M-CSF are under intensive clinical investigation.

IL-3, a T-cell-derived cytokine, promotes the proliferation and differentiation of multipotential stem cells and of committed progenitor cells in vitro. In vivo studies in primates have shown that IL-3 was a poor hematopoietic stimulus. However, when IL-3 treatment was followed by low-dose administration of GM-CSF, a profound increase in neutrophils, monocytes, eosinophils, reticulocytes and also in platelets was observed [32–34]. Based on these results, it was suggested that IL-3 may expand the GM-CSF-sensitive population of progenitors. The first clinical trial with IL-3 in tumor patients with normal hematopoiesis and in patients with bone marrow failure was published recently [35]. This treatment induced a multilineage hematopoietic response, the most promising response being the increase in platelets and reticulocytes. In contrast to treatment of patients with GM-CSF or G-CSF, the rise in leukocyte counts induced by IL-3 was delayed and first seen at days 10–15 after initiation of IL-3 treatment. This delayed response is consistent with the concept that IL-3 exerts its main action at the level of multipotent and committed pro-

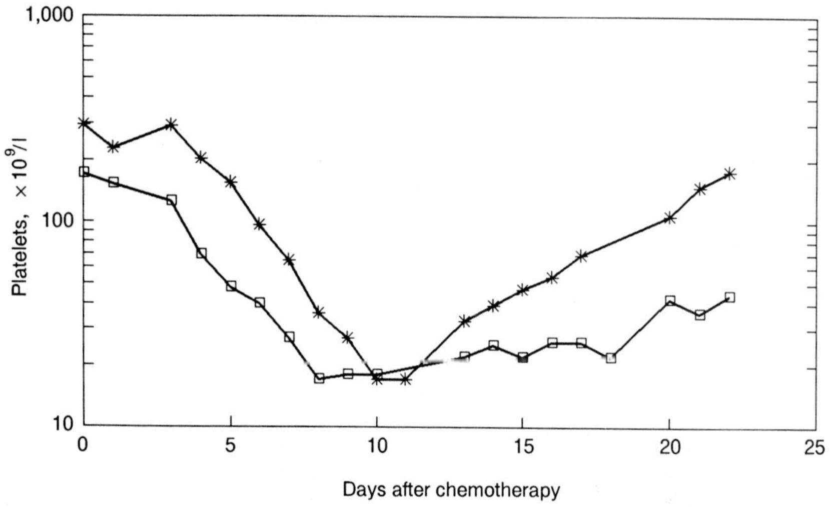

Fig. 1. Platelet recovery in a heavily pretreated patient with Hodgkin's disease, treated twice with a high-dose chemotherapy (cyclo-phosphamide 1,600 mg/m^2, VP 16, 500 mg/m^2, cisplatin 50 mg/m^2) followed by sequential subcutaneous administration of either recombinant human GM-CSF (250 μg/m^2 d1–15) (□) or recombinant human IL-3 (250 μg/m^2 d1–d5) and recombinant human GM-CSF (250 μg/m^2 d6–d15) (*), respectively.

genitor cells and not at the level of myeloid precursor cells in the bone marrow.

IL-3 treatment was well tolerated with the exception of mild to moderate fever and headache, and acrocyanosis and neck stiffness at higher doses.

In order to accelerate hematopoiesis after myelosuppressive chemotherapy, some patients are currently treated at our institution with a sequential subcutaneous administration of IL-3 and GM-CSF. Preliminary results indicate that recovery of platelets was shortened for several days, as compared to patients treated with GM-CSF alone (fig. 1) [36]. In addition, the sequential application of IL-3 and GM-CSF in these patients induced a dramatic increase in CD34-positive cells as well as in all peripheral blood progenitor cells (as analyzed by culture assays), suggesting that these cells might be used as peripheral blood stem cell graft after high-dose intensification chemotherapy.

GM-CSF, a glycoprotein of 14–35 kD, was purified from a HTLV-II infected T-lymphoblast cell line [37]. Its human genomic clone has been isolated and the GM-CSF gene localized to chromosome 5q21–32 [38, 39]. This gene is localized together with the genes for IL-3, M-CSF and the receptor for M-CSF (c-fms proto-oncogene) on a small segment of chromosome 5.

Under normal conditions, GM-CSF is not expressed constitutively, but following activation, different cell types including T cells, endothelial cells, fibroblasts and monocytes express GM-CSF mRNA [40–43]. High-affinity GM-CSF receptors have been identified on mature neutrophils, monocytes, eosinophils, CML cells, AML cells and on several myeloid leukemic cell lines [18, 44, 45]. Interestingly, GM-CSF receptors have also been identified on non-hematopoietic cell lines including small cell lung carcinoma and melanoma [46].

The biological activities of GM-CSF are more restricted when compared to IL-3. In vitro, it supportes the proliferation of neutrophils, macrophage and eosinophilic colonies and, together with EPO, it also acts on erythroid progenitors [47]. In addition, GM-CSF was shown to have megakaryocytic activity in vitro [48–50] and augments megakaryocyte colony stimulation by IL-3 [51]. GM-CSF also induces a variety of functional changes in mature target cells, such as increased arachidonic acid release [52], enhanced phagocytic and cytotoxic activity [53], increased expression of cell-cell adhesion molecules [54], stimulation of ADCC by macrophages [55], augmentation of oxygen radical release [56] or increased production of other cytokines [57–59].

In vivo studies with GM-CSF were initially performed in primates after total body irradiation and autologous bone marrow transplantation. In these studies, GM-CSF was shown to stimulate hematopoiesis and to shorten the period of neutropenia and thrombopenia [60–62]. Given subcutaneously, GM-CSF treatment resulted in a dose-dependent increase in granulocytes, monocytes and lymphocytes [63]. These data led to clinical trials in tumor patients following myelosuppressive chemotherapy, where GM-CSF was expected to decrease the incidence and severity of bacterial infections. This could be shown in various studies where the neutrophil nadir was significantly shortened and patients were protected from febrile events and severe infections [64–66]. In the setting of autologous bone marrow transplantation, earlier hematopoietic reconstitution was also shown to occur with GM-CSF [67–70].

Side effects of GM-CSF at doses of $< 250\ \mu g/m^2$ s.c. were mild, consisting of occasional low-grade fever, bone pain and weakness. Other adverse effects like a short-lived dyspnea was seen only occasionally in patients with elevated granulocytes and was most likely due to activation of neutrophils and accumulation in pulmonary circulation.

G-CSF, which is primarily produced by monocytes, fibroblasts and endothelial cells [41, 43, 71), has been purified by Welte et al. [72] and molecularly cloned [73, 74]. It is encoded by a single gene located on chromosome 17q11–21 [75]. G-CSF shows a significant homology with interleukin-6 [76].

In vitro, G-CSF induces granulocyte lineage specific colony growth [74], acts synergistically with IL-3 to stimulate megakaryocyte colonies and blast cell colonies and causes functional activation of peripheral neutrophils including enhancement of chemotaxis, antibody-dependent cell-mediated cytotoxicity and expression of FMLP and surface Fc receptors for immunoglobulins [77–79].

Similar to GM-CSF, clinical studies have demonstrated the capacity of this hormone to increase bone marrow cellularity and peripheral blood neutrophil counts in chemotherapy-induced neutropenia as well as following autologous bone marrow transplantation [80–84]. Toxicities in G-CSF trials have been minimal, essentially being limited to bone pain.

M-CSF is a lineage-specific hematopoietin that stimulates proliferation and supports differentiation and survival of cells of the mononuclear phagocyte system. It is a 70- to 90-kD homodimeric glycoprotein [85–87] synthesized by fibroblasts, endothelial cells, monocytes and macrophages in response to other cytokines or additional stimuli [88, 89]. M-CSF mRNA is transcribed from a single gene that maps together with other growth factor genes to the long arm of chromosome 5 at band q33.1 [90]. M-CSF induces formation of pure macrophage colonies in vitro and potentiates the ability of mature mononuclear phagocytes to perform their effector functions by enhancing their ability to kill infectious microorganisms [91] or tumor cells [92, 93] and by regulating release of macrophage cytokines, such as interferon-alpha, TNF-alpha, IL-1 or G-CSF [94, 95], as well as inflammatory signals, such as prostaglandins, oxygen radicals, and plasminogen activator [96, 97]. M-CSF exerts its pleiotropic effects by binding to a single class of high-affinity receptors [98] which is a growth factor receptor that exhibits ligand-induced tyrosine-specific protein kinase activity [99].

In animal models, M-CSF induced a dose-dependent peripheral monocytosis, neutrophilia, and lymphopenia. The monocytosis peaked at about 30 h, with a seven- to eightfold increase in monocytes and promonocytes. A monocytopenia reaching a nadir at 15 min preceded monocytosis, suggesting that M-CSF activated circulating monocytes and caused intravascular margination. The neutrophilia and lymphopenia may reflect indirect effects mediated by the release of other monokines [100]. Clinical studies with natural human M-CSF were published recently by Motoyoshi et al. [101a], indicating that human M-CSF accelerates the production of neutrophils and interestingly also of platelets after anticancer chemotherapy and bone marrow transplantation. In addition, it was shown that natural M-CSF improved the survival rate after bone marrow transplantation. To date, only preliminary studies with recombinant human M-CSF have been published [101b]; a phase I/II trial has just started at our institution.

Stimulation of Hematopoiesis in Primary Bone Marrow Failure

CSFs are very promising molecules for the stimulation of hematopoiesis in some primary marrow failure syndromes, such as cyclic and idiopathic neutropenia or congenital agranulocytosis (Kostman's syndrome).

In patients with congenital agranulocytosis, G-CSF induced an increase in neutrophil counts, accompanied by the resolution of preexisting chronic infections [102, 103]. In patients with cyclic or idiopathic neutropenia G-CSF was also shown to be effective [104, 105].

Since IL-3 acts on pluripotent stem cells as well as on restricted progenitor cells, IL-3 might be of value in the treatment of stem cell disorders. Recently, IL-3 was shown to induce a multilineage response in patients with aplasic anemia, though the overall response was much less impressive as compared to patients with residual hematopoiesis [106]. GM-CSF seems not to be effective in patients with severe aplastic anemia [107–109].

CSFs in the Treatment of Acute Myelogenous Leukemia and Myelodysplasia

The available data on the efficacy of CSFs in solid tumors following intensive cytotoxic chemotherapy suggest that these factors may also be useful to accelerate neutrophil regeneration after successful induction chemotherapy in AML, when the leukemic cells are highly reduced and normal progenitors are available to respond [110]. It was shown that these factors effectively can promote recovery of hematopoiesis after chemotherapy without evidence of GM-CSF induced leukemic blast-cell resistance [111]. As G-CSF, GM-CSF and IL-3 are able to recruit leukemic progenitors into chemotherapy-sensitive cell-cycle phases [112, 113], these factors are now under investigation in several clinical trials using a combined therapy of GM-CSF with a standard cytotoxic chemotherapy regimen in AML (daunorubicin plus cytosine-arabinoside) [114].

In patients with myelodysplastic syndromes, G-, GM-CSF and IL-3 induced increased numbers of neutrophils and also an increase in bone marrow cellularity, whereas platelet counts and red cells increased only in a very small number of patients [115–118]. At higher doses of GM-CSF (>500 μg/m^2), several investigators observed an increase in the number of circulating and bone marrow blasts, indicating that GM-CSF can stimulate the proliferation of human leukemic blasts in vivo [116]. These observations, however, form the basis of new treatment strategies in these patients in an effort to recruit quiescent cells by GM-CSF which would then be targets for subsequent cycle-specific cytotoxic chemotherapy [114].

Expansion and Recruitment of Circulating Progenitor Cells

Autologous blood stem cells have been used successfully to rescue animals from otherwise lethal marrow aplasia induced by radiation or chemotherapy [120]. In humans, increased numbers of hematopoietic progenitor cells can also be detected in the peripheral blood following transient myelosuppressive chemotherapy [121]. Recently, GM-CSF was shown to further increase the pool of circulating progenitor cells with or without prior chemotherapy, thus enhancing the amount of cells possibly being harvested by leukapheresis [122–124]. These cells are then able to repopulate the bone marrow as an alternative to autologous bone marrow transplantation [125] or might be used for rescue after high-dose intensification chemotherapy [126].

Activation of Effector Cell Function

As CSFs are known to induce a variety of functional changes in mature effector cells (e.g. neutrophils or macrophages), CSFs might be useful in the treatment of infectious diseases, leukocyte dysfunctions or in the stimulation of monocyte/macrophage-mediated anticancer effects.

For example, M-CSF was shown to be effective in patients with invasive fungal infections post bone marrow transplantation since M-CSF enhances the fungicidal activity of macrophages [127].

In addition, CSFs might be effective in the treatment of leukopenic patients with AIDS [128] or in improving AIDS patients' tolerance to both AZT and antibiotics that are required to fight infections [129].

As macrophages are also known to act in host defense against tumor growth and metastasis, particularily after activation with endotoxin or cytokines [130], and as M-CSF was shown to enhance ADCC [93, 131], treatment with M-CSF was suggested to induce antitumor effects in vivo. Treatment of monkeys with recombinant M-CSF indeed resulted in an increased antitumor ADCC [132]. This observation would support the design of combined growth factor and antibody trials.

Future Prospects of CSF

Animal trials have documented superadditive responses of the combined application of CSFs. These findings supported the combination therapy of CSFs in patients. We started to combine IL-3 plus GM-CSF in a sequential mode at our institution; preliminary results demonstrate its efficacy concerning platelet recovery after chemotherapy as compared to GM-CSF alone (fig. 1). Another approach might be the combined therapy of late-acting CSFs (e.g. G-CSF) with CSFs predominantly acting on early progenitors, such as IL-1 [133] or IL-6 [134]. The single administration of IL-1 in animals enhanced the resistance of normal and granulocytopenic mice to infections and was able to protect mice from irradiation-associated neutropenia. In tumor-bearing mice, IL-α administration had a chemoprotective effect and allowed enhanced therapeutic efficacy by permitting the use of increased doses of chemotherapeutic drugs [135].

In addition to its activity as a hematopoetin, IL-1 displays several regulatory functions in the immune response including cytotoxicity and induction of the acute-phase reaction. Therefore IL-1 might be a potent stimulator not only of hematopoiesis but also acts as a mediator molecule for the induction of antitumor effects. Preliminary data with IL-1 have been published recently; we are now going to start a phase I study of IL-1β in patients with advanced malignancies.

IL-6 seems to be one of the most promising cytokines with thrombopoietic activities. Asano et al. [136] and Welte et al. [137] were the first to describe this activity in monkeys. Moreover, Welte et al. [138] have recently shown a similar increase in platelets when monkeys were given leukemia inhibitory factor [138]. Our ongoing studies indicate that megakaryopoiesis is regulated by a specific CSF [139]; we have therefore initiated the biochemical characterization of this putative Meg-CSF.

The clinical role of the stem cell factor, a factor which was shown to be the c-kit ligand [140, 141], and to synergize with CSFs and EPO [142], has to be defined. First in vivo studies in baboons have been published and demonstrated the proliferation and maturation of cells of multiple lineages. This factor might be of crucial importance concerning hematopoietic stem cell transplantation.

Up to now, the significant reduction of chemotherapy-associated morbidity by CSFs has to be considered as a major goal in cancer therapy, but it remains to be determined whether this new dimension will be primarily of palliative benefit, or whether the options for increased dose intensity protocols will result in an increase in long-term survival in some patient groups.

References

1 Bradley TR, Metcalf D: The growth of mouse bone marrow cells in vitro. Aust J Exp Biol Med Sci 1966;44:287–299.

2 Ichikawa Y, Pluznik DH, Sachs L: In vitro control of the development of macrophage and granulocyte colonies. Proc Natl Acad Sci USA 1966;56:488–495.

3 Spivac JL: The mechanisms of action of erythropoietin. Int J Cell Cloning 1986;4:139–166.

4 Eaves CJ, Eaves AC: Erythropoietin dose-response curves for three classes of erythroid progenitors in normal human marrow and in patients with polycythemia vera. Blood 1978;52:1196–1210.

5 Koury ST, Bondurant MC, Koury MJ: Localization of erythropoietin synthesizing cells in murine kidneys by in situ hybridization. Blood 1988;71:524–527.

6 Lacombe C, da Silva JL, Bruneval P, Fournier JG, Wendling F, et al: Peritubular cells are the site of erythropoietin synthesis in the murine hypoxic kidney. J Clin Invest 1988;81:620–623.

7 Erslev AJ, Caro J, Kansu E, Silver R: Renal and extrarenal erythropoietin production in anaemic rats. Br J Haemat 1980;45:65.

8 Rich IN, Heit W, Kubanek B: Extrarenal erythropoietin production by macrophages. Blood 1982;60:1007.

9 Miyake T, Kung CK, Goldwasser E: Purification of human erythropoietin. J Biol Chem 1977;252:5564–5568.

10 Law ML, Cai C-H, Lin F-K, Wei A, Huang S-Z, Hartz J-H, Morse H, Lin C-H, Jones C, Kao F-T: Chromosomal assignment of the human erythropoietin gene and its DNA polymorphism. Proc Natl Acad Sci USA 1986;83:6920–6924.

11 D'Andrea AD, Lodish HF, Wong GG: Expression cloning of the murine erythropoietin receptor. Cell 1989;57:277.

12 Winkelmann JC, Penny LA, Deaven LL, Forget BG, Jenkins RB: The gene for the human erythropoietin receptor: Analysis of the coding sequence and assignment to chromosome 19p. Blood 1990;76:24–30.

13 Jones SS, D'Andrea AD, Haines LL, Wong GG: Human erythropoietin receptor: cloning, expression and biologic characterization. Blood 1990;76:31–35.

14 D'Andrea AD, Fasman GD, Lodish HF: Erythropoietin receptor and interleukin-2 receptor β chain: A new receptor family. Cell 1989;58:1023.

15 Itoh N, Yonehara S, Schreurs J, Gorman DM, Maruyama K, et al: Cloning of an interleukin-3 receptor gene: A member of a distinct receptor gene family. Science 1990;247:324.

16 Mosley B, Beckmann MP, March CJ, Idzerda RL, Gimpel SD, et al: The murine interleukin-4 receptor: molecular cloning and characterization of secreted and membrane bound forms. Cell 1989;59:335.

17 Urdal DL, Idzerda RL, Beckmann MP, Cosman D, March CK, Park LS: Receptors of hematopoietic growth factors; in Mertelsmann R, Herrmann F (eds): Hematopoietic Growth Factors in Clinical Applications. New York, Dekker, 1989.

18 Gearing DP, King JA, Gough NM, Nicola NA: Expression cloning of a receptor for human granulocyte-macrophage colony-stimulating factor. EMBO J 1989;8:3667.

19 Adamson JW: The promise of recombinant human erythropoietin. Seminars in Hematology 1989;26:5–8.

20 Eschbach JW, Egrie JC, Downing MR, Browne JK, Adamson JW: Correction of the anemia of end-stage renal disease with recombinant human erythropoietin. N Engl J Med 1987;316:73–80.

21 Eschbach JW, Kelly MR, Haley NR, Abels RI, Adamson JW: Treatment of the anemia of progressive renal failure with recombinant human erythropoietin. N Engl J Med 1989;321:158–163.

22 Lim VS, DeGowin RL, Zavala D, Kirchner PT, Abels R, Perry P, Fangman J: Recombinant human erythropoietin treatment in pre-dialysis patients. Ann Intern Med 1989;110:108–114.

23 Ludwig H, Fritz E, Kotzmann H, Höcker P, Gisslinger H, Bar-

nas U: Erythropoietin treatment of anemia associated with multiple myeloma. N Engl J Med 1990;322:1693–1699.
24 Oster W, Herrmann F, Gamm H, Zeile G, Lindemann A, Müller G, Brune T, Kraemer HP, Mertelsmann R: Erythropoietin (EPO) for the treatment of anemia of malignancy associated with neoplastic bone marrow infiltration. J Clin Oncol 1990;6:956–962.
25 Fischl M, Galpin JE, Levine JD, Groopmann JE, Henry DH, Kennedy P, et al: Recombinant human erythropoietin for patients with AIDS treated with zidovudine. N Engl J Med 1990;322:1488–1493.
26 Means RT, Olsen NJ, Krantz SB, et al: Treatment of the anemia of rheumatoid arthritis with recombinant human erythropoietin: Clinical and in vitro studies. Arthritis Rheum 1989;32:638–642.
27 Oster W, Herrmann F, Cicco A, Gamm H, Zeile G, Brune T, Lindemann A, Schulz G, Mertelsmann R: Erythropoietin prevents chemotherapy-induced anemia. Blut 1990;60:88–92.
28 Miller CB, Platanias LC, Ratain MJ, et al: A phase I/II trial of erythropoietin in the treatment of chemotherapy-induced anemia in patients with cancer. Proc Am Soc Clin Oncol 1990;9:194.
29 Henry DH, Rudnick SA, Bryant E, et al: Preliminary report of two double-blind, placebo-controlled studies using recombinant human erythropoietin in the anemia associated with cancer (abstract). Blood 1988;73:suppl 52.
30 Miller CB, Jones RJ, Piantadosi S, Abeloff MD, Spivak JL: Decreased erythropoietin response in patients with the anemia of cancer. N Engl J Med 1990;322:1689–1692.
31 Goodnough LT, Rudnick S, Price T, Ballas SK, Collins ML, et al: Increased preoperative collection of autologous blood with recombinant human erythropoietin therapy. N Engl J Med 1989;321:1163–1168.
32 Leary AG, Yang YC, Clark SC, et al: Recombinant gibbon interleukin-3 supports formation of human multilineage colonies and blast cell colonies in culture: Comparison with recombinant human granulocyte-macrophage colony-stimulating factor. Blood 1987;70:1343–1348.
33 Donahue RE, Seehra J, Metzger M, Lefebvre D, Rock B, et al: Human interleukin-3 and GM-CSF act synergistically in stimulating hematopoiesis in primates. Science 1988;241:1820.
34 Krumwieh D, Seiler FR: In vivo effects of recombinant colony stimulating factors on hematopoiesis in cynamolgus monkeys. Transplant Proc 1989;21:379.
35 Ganser A, Lindemann, A, Seipelt G, Ottmann OG, Herrmann F, et al: Effects of recombinant human interleukin-3 in patients with normal hematopoiesis and in patients with bone marrow failure. Blood 1990;76:666–676.
36 Kanz L, Brugger W, Bross KJ, Mertelsmann R: Combination of hematopoietic growth factors. Current status and future prospects. Br J Haematol, in press.
37 Gasson JC, Weisbart RH, Kaufmann SE, Clark SC, et al: Science 1984;226:1339–1342.
38 Wong GG, Witek JS, Temple PA, et al: Human GM-CSF: Molecular cloning of the cDNA and purification of the natural and recombinant proteins. Science 1985;228:810–815.
39 Huebner K, Isobe M, Croce CM, Golde W, Kaufmann SE, Gasson JC: The human gene encoding GM-CSF is a 5q29–32, the chromosome region deleted in the 5q-anomaly. Science 1985;230:1282–1285.
40 Herrmann F, Oster W, Meuer SC, Klein K, Lindemann A, Mertelsmann R: Interleukin-1 stimulates T lymphocytes to produce GM-CSF. J Clin Invest 1988;81:1415–1418.
41 Herrmann F, Cannistra SA, Griffin JD: T-cell monocyte interactions in the production of humoral factors regulating human granulopoiesis in vitro. J Immunol 1986;136:2856–2861.
42 Sieff CA, Niemeyer CM, Mentzer SJ, Faller DV: Interleukin-1, tumor necrosis factor, and the production of colony-stimulating factors by cultured mesenchymal cells. Blood 1987;72:1316–1323.
43 Zsebo KM, Yuschenkoff VN, Schiffer S, et al: Vascular endothelial cells and granulopoiesis: Interleukin-1 stimulates release of G-CSF and GM-CSF. Blood 1988;71:99–103.
44 Gasson JC, Kaufman SE, Weisbart RH, et al: High-affinity binding of GM-CSF to normal and leukemic human myeloid cells. Proc Natl Acad Sci USA 1986;83:669–673.
45 Di Persio JF, Billing P, Kaufman SE, Eghtesady P, et al: Characterization of the human GM-CSF receptor. J Biol Chem 1988;263:1834–1841.
46 Baldwin GC, Gasson JC, Kaufman SE, et al: Non-hematopoietic tumor cells express functional GM-CSF receptors. Blood 1989;73:1033–1037.
47 Sieff CA: Hematopoietic growth factors. J Clin Invest 1987;79:1549–1557.
48 Sieff CA, Niemeyer CM, Nathan DC, et al: Stimulation of human hematopoietic colony formation by recombinant gibbon multi-colony-stimulating factor or interleukin-3. J Clin Invest 1987;80:818–823.
49 Mazur EM, Cohen JL, Wong GG, Clark SC: Modest stimulatory effect of recombinant human GM-CSF on colony growth from peripheral blood human megakaryocyte progenitor cells. Exp Hematol 1987;15:1128–1123.
50 Messner HA, Yamasaki Km Jamal N, et al: Growth of human hemopoietic colonies in response to recombinant gibbon interleukin-3: comparison with human recombinant granulocyte and granulocyte-macrophage colony-stimulating factors. Proc Natl Acad Sci USA 1987;84:6765–6769.
51 Robinson BE, McGrath HE, Quesenberry PJ: Recombinant murine granulocyte macrophage colony-stimulating factor has megakaryocytic colony-stimulating activity and augments megakaryocyte colony stimulation by interleukin-3. J Clin Invest 1987;79:1648–1652.
52 Di Persio JF, Billing P, William R, et al: Human GM-CSF and other cytokines prime human neutrophils for enhanced arachidonic acid release and leukotriene B4 synthesis. J Immunol 1988;140:5315–5322.
53 Fleischmann J, Golde DW, Weisbart RH, Gasson JC: GM-CSF enhances phagocytosis of bacteria by human neutrophils. Blood 1986;68:708–711.
54 Arnaout MA, Wang EA, Clark SC, Sieff CA: Human recombinant GM-CSF increases cell-to-cell adhesion and surface expression of adhesion-promoting surface glycoproteins on mature granulocytes. J Clin Invest 1986;78:587–601.
55 Grabstein KH, Urdal DL, Tushinsi RJ, Mochizuki DY, et al: Induction of macrophage tumoricidal activity by GM-CSF. Science 1986;32:506–508.
56 Nathan CF: Respiratory burst in adherent human neutrophils: Triggering by GM-CSF and G-CSF. Blood 1989;73:301–306.
57 Lindemann A, Riedel D, Oster W, Meuer SC, Blohm D, Mertelsmann R, Herrmann F: GM-CSF induces secretion of in-

terleukin-1 by polymorphonuclear neutrophils. J Immunol 1988;140:837–839.
58 Oster W, Lindemann A, Mertelsmann R, Herrmann F: Granulocyte-macrophage colony-stimulating factor (CSF) and multilineage CSF recruit human monocytes to express granulocyte CSF. Blood 1989;73:64–67.
59 Lindemann A, Riedel D, Oster W, Ziegler-Heitbrock HW, Mertelsmann R, Herrmann F: Granulocyte-macrophage colony-stimulating factor induces cytokine secretion by human polymorphonuclear leukocytes. J Clin Invest 1989;83:1308–1312.
60 Donahue RE, Wang EA, Stone DK, et al: Stimulation of hemopoiesis in primates by continuous infusion of recombinant GM-CSF. Nature 1986;321:872–875.
61 Nienhuis AW, Donahue RE, Karisson S, et al: Recombinant human GM-CSF shortens the period of neutropenia after autologous bone marrow transplantation in a primate model. J Clin Invest 1987;80:573–577.
62 Monroy RL, Skelly TJ, Mac Vittie TA, et al: The effect of recombinant GM-CSF on the recovery of monkeys transplanted with autologous bone marrow. Blood 1987;70:1696–1699.
63 Nayer P, Lam C, Obenaus H, et al: Recombinant human GM-CSF induces leukocytosis and activates peripheral blood polymorphonuclear neutrophils in nonhuman primates. Blood 1987;70:206–213.
64 Antmann KS, Griffin JD, Elias A, Socinski MA, et al: Effect of recombinant human GM-CSF of chemotherapy-induced myelosuppression. N Engl J Med 1988;319:593–598.
65 Herrmann F, Schulz G, Lindemann A, Meyenburg W, Oster W, Krumwieh D, Mertelsmann R: Hematopoietic responses in patients with advanced malignancy treated with recombinant human granulocyte-macrophage colony-stimulating factor. J Clin Oncol 1989;7:159–167.
66 Herrmann F, Schulz G, Wieser M, Kolbe K, Nicolay U, Noack M, Lindemann A, Mertelsmann R: Effect of GM-CSF on neutropenia and related morbidity induced by myelotoxic chemotherapy. Am J Med 1990;88:619–624.
67 Brandt SJ, Peters WP, Atwater SK, Kurtzberg J, Borowitz MJ, et al: Effect of recombinant human granulocyte-macrophage colony-stimulating factor on hematopoietic reconstitution after high-dose chemotherapy and autologous bone marrow transplantation. N Engl J Med 1988;318:869–876.
68 Peters WP: The effect of recombinant human colony-stimulating factors on hematopoietic reconstitution following autologous bone marrow transplantation. Semin Hematol 1989;26:18–23.
69 Peters WP, Atwater S, Kurtzberg J: The use of recombinant human granulocyte macrophage colony-stimulating factor in autologous bone marrow transplantation; in Gale R, Champlin R (eds): Bone Marrow Transplantation: Current Controversies. New York, Liss, 1989, pp 595–606.
70 Nemunaitis J, Singer JW, Buckner CD, Durnam D, Epstein C, Hill R, Storb R, Thomas Ed, Appelbaum FR: Use of recombinant human GM-CSF in graft failure after bone marrow transplantation. Blood 1990;76:245–253.
71 Kaushansky K, Lin N, Adamson JW: Interleukin-1 stimulates fibroblast to synthesize GM-CSF and G-CSF. J Clin Invest 1988;81:87–92.
72 Welte K, Platzer E, Lu L, Gabrilove JL, Levi E, Mertelsmann R, Moore MAS: Purification and biological characterization of human pluripotent hematopoietic colony-stimulating factor. Proc Natl Acad Sci USA 1985;82:1526–1530.
73 Nagata S, Tsuchiya M, Asano S, Kaziro Y, Yamazaki T, Yamamozo O, Hirata N, Kubota N, Oheda H, Nomura H, Ono M: Molecular cloning and expression of cDNA for human granulocyte colony-stimulating factor. Nature 1986;319:415–418.
74 Souza LM, Boone TC, Gabrilove JL, Lai PH, Zsebo KM, Murdock DC, et al: Rcombinant human granulocyte colony-stimulating factor: Effects on normal and leukemic myeloid cells. Science 1986;232:61–65.
75 Simmers RN, Webber LM, Shannon MF, Garson OM, Wong MA, Sutherland GR: Localization of the G-CSF gene on chromosome 17 proximal to the breakpoint in the t(15;17) in acute promyelocytic leukemia. Blood 1987;70:330–332.
76 Hirano T, Yasukawa K, Harada H, Tag T, Watanabe Y, et al: Complementary DNA for a novel human interleukin (BSF-2) that induces B lymphocytes to induce immunoglobulin. Nature 1986;324:73.
77 Platzer E, Oez K, Welte K, Sandler A, Gabrilove JL, Mertelsman R, Moore MA, Kalden JR: Human pluripotent hematopoietic colony stimulating factor; activities on human and murine cells. Immunobiology 1987;172:185–193.
78 Platzer E, Welte K, Gabrilov JC, Harris P, et al: Biological activities of a human pluripotent hemopoietic colony-stimulating factor on normal and leukemic cells. J Exp Med 1985;162:1788.
79 Weisbart RH, Kacen A, Schuh A, Golde DW: GM-CSF induces human neutrophil IgA-mediated phagocytosis by an IgA Fc receptor activation mechanism. Nature 1988;332:647.
80 Sheridan WP, Wolf M, Lusk J, et al: G-CSF and neutrophil recovery after high-dose chemotherapy and autologous bone marrow transplantation. Lancet 1989;ii:891–895.
81 Bronchud M, Scarfte JH, Thatcher N, Crowther D, Souza LM, Alton NK, Testa NG, Dexter TM: Phase I/II study of recombinant human granulocyte colony-stimulating factor in patients receiving intensive chemotherapy for small cell lung cancer. Br J Cancer 1987;56:809–813.
82 Gabrilove JL, Jakubowski A, Scher H, Sternberg C, Wong G, et al: Effect of granulocyte colony-stimulating factor on neutropenia and associated morbidity due to chemotherapy or transitional cell carcinoma of the urothelium. N Engl J Med 1988;318:1414–1422.
83 Lindemann A, Herrmann F, Oster W, Meyenburg W, Haffneer P, Souza L, Mertelsmann R: Hematologic effects of recombinant human granulocyte colony-stimulating factor in patients with malignancy. Blood 1989;8:2644–2651.
84 Morstyn G, Campbell L, Souza LM, Alton NK, Keech J, Green M, et al: Effect of granulocyte colony-stimulating factor on neutropenia induced by cytotoxic chemotherapy. Lancet 1988; i:667–672.
85 Stanley ER, Guilbert LJ, Tushinski RJ, Bartelemz SH: CSF-1. A mononuclear phagocyte lineage-specific hematopoietic growth factor. J Cell Biochem 1983;21:151.
86 Kawasaki ES, Ladner MB, Wang AM, et al: Molecular cloning of a cDNA encoding human macrophage specific colony stimulating factor (CSF-1). Science 1985;230:291–296.
87 Wong GG, Temple PA, Leary AC, et al: Human CSF-1: Molecular cloning and expression of 4 kb cDNA encoding the human urinary protein. Science 1987;235:1504–1508.
88 Oster W, Lindemann A, Horn S, Mertelsmann R, Herrmann F: TNF alpha but not TNF beta induces secretion of colony stim-

ulating factor for macrophages by human monocytes. Blood 1987;70:1409.
89 Rambaldi A, Young DC, Griffin JD: Expression of the CSF-1 gene by human monocytes. Blood 1987;69:1409.
90 Pettenati MJ, Le Beau MM, Lemons RS, Shima EA, et al: Assignment of CSF-1 to 5q311.1: Evidence for clustering of genes of the long arm of chromosome 5 in myeloid disorders. Proc Natl Acad Sci USA 1987;84:2970.
91 Lee MT, Warren MK: CSF-1 induced resistance to viral infection in murine macrophages. J Immunol 1987;138:3019.
92 Ralph P, Nakoinz I: Stimulation of macrophage tumoricidal activity by the growth and differentiation factor CSF-1. Cell Immunol 1987;105:270.
93 Munn DH, Cheung NK: Antibody-dependent antitumor cytotoxicity by human monocytes cultured with recombinant M-CSF. J Exp Med 1989;170:511–526.
94 Moore RN, Larsen HS, Horohov DS, Rouse BT: Endogenous regulation of macrophage proliferative expansion by colony stimulating factor-induced interferon. Science 1984;223:178.
95 Warren MK, Ralph P: Macrophage growth factor CSF-1 stimulates human monocyte production of interferon, tumor necrosis factor, and colony stimulating activity. J Immunol 1986; 137:2281.
96 Kurland JI, Bockman R: Prostaglandin E production by human blood monocytes and mouse peritoneal macrophages. J Exp Med 1978;147:952.
97 Wing EJ, Ampel NM, Waheed A, Shadduck RK: M-CSF enhances the capacity of murine macrophages to secrete oxygen reduction products. J Immunol 1985;135:2052.
98 Rettenmier CW; Sacca R, Furman WL, et al: Expression of the human c-fms proto-oncogene product (CSF-1 receptor) on peripheral blood mononuclear cells and choriocarcinoma cell lines. J Clin Invest 1986;77:1740.
99 Hanks SK, Quinn AM, Hunter T: The protein kinase family: Conserved features and deduced phylogeny of the catalytic domains. Science 1988;241:42.
100 Ulich TR, del Castillo J, Watson LR, Yin S, Garnick MG: In vivo hematologic effects of recombinant human M-CSF. Blood 1990;75:846–850.
101_a Motoyoshi K, Takaku F: Human monocytic colony-stimulating factor (hM CSF), phase I/II studies; in Mertelsmann R, Herrmann F (eds): Hematopoietic growth factors in clinical applications. New York, Dekker, 1990, pp 161–175.
101_b Bajorin DA, Jakibowski A, Cody B, Chapman P, et al: Phase I trial of recombinant human M-CSF in patients with melanoma. Blood 1989;74(suppl 1):323a.
102 Bonilla MA, Gillio AP, Ruggiero M, Kernan NA, Brochstein JA, et al: Effects of recombinant human G-CSF on the neutropenia in patients with congenital agranulocytosis. N Engl J Med 1989;320:1574–1580.
103 Welte K, Zeidler C, Reiter A, Müller W, Odenwald E, Souza L, Riehm H: Differential effects of GM-CSF and G-CSF in children with severe congenital neutropenia. Blood 1990;75: 1056–1063.
104 Hammond WP, Price TH, Souza LM, Dale DC: Treatment of cyclic neutropenia with granulocyte colony-stimulating factor. N Engl J Med 1989;320:1306–1311.
105 Jakubowski AA, Souza L, Kelly F, Fain K, Budman D, et al: Effects of granulocyte colony-stimulating factor in a patient with idiopathic neutropenia. N Engl J Med 1989;320:38–42.
106 Ganser A, Lindemann A, Seipelt G, Ottmann OG, Eder M, et al: Effects of recombinant human interleukin-3 in aplastic anemia. Blood 1990;76:1287–1292.
107 Antin JH, Smith BR, Holmes W, et al: Phase I/II study of recombinant human GM-CSF in aplastic and myelodysplastic syndrome. Blood 1988;72:705–713.
108 Champlin RE, Nimer SD, Ireland P, Oette DH, Golde DW: Treatment of refractory aplastic anemia with recombinant human granulocyte-macrophage colony-stimulating factor. Blood 1989;73:694–699.
109 Nissen C, Tichelli A, Gratwohl A, Speck B, Milne A, Gordon-Smith EC, Schaedelin J: Failure of recombinant human granulocyte-macrophage colony-stimulating factor therapy in aplastic anemia patients with severe neutropenia. Blood 1988;72:2045–2047.
110 Ohno R, Tomonaga M, Kobayashi T, Kanamaru A, Shirakawa S, Masaoka T, et al: Effect of G-CSF after intensive induction therapy in relapsed or refractory acute leukemia. N Engl J Med 1990;323:871–877.
111 Büchner T, Hiddemann W, Koenigsmann M, Zuehlsdorf M, Woermann B, Boeckmann A, Freire EA, Innig G, et al: GM-CSF for acute leukemias in aplasia and at high risk of early death; in Mertelsmann R, Herrmann F (eds): Hematopoietic Growth Factors in Clinical Applications. New York, Dekker, 1990, pp 291–301.
112 Tafuri A, Andreeff M: Cell kinetic modulation of hematological malignancies by cytokines: Recruitment therapy to overcome cytokinetic resistance; in Mertelsmann R, Herrmann F (eds): Hematopoietic Growth Factors in Clinical Applications. New York, Dekker, 1990, pp 381–399.
113 Brach M, Klein H, Platzer E, Mertelsmann R, Herrmann F: Effect of interleukin-3 on cytosin arabinoside-mediated cytotoxicity of leukemic myeloblasts. Exp Hematol 1990;18:748–753.
114 Bettelheim P, Muhm M, Geissler K, Gorischek C, Hinterberger W, Speiser W, Sunder-Plassmann G, Valent P, Lechner K, Andreeff M, Haimi J, Haas O, Maurer D, Schulz G: GM-CSF during remission induction for acute myelogenous leukemia; in Mertelsmann R, Herrmann F (eds): Hematopoietic Growth Factors in Clinical Applications. New York, Dekker, 1990, pp 401–420.
115 Ganser A, Seipelt G, Lindemann A, Ottmann OG, Falk S, Eder M, et al: Effects of recombinant human interleukin-3 in patients with myelodysplastic syndromes. Blood 1990;76:455–462.
116 Herrmann F, Lindemann A, Klein H, Lübbert M, Schulz G, Mertelsmann R: Effect of recombinant human GM-CSF in patients with myelodysplastic syndrome with excess blasts. Leukemia 1989;3:335–338.
117 Vadhan-Raj S, Keating M, LeMaistre A, Hittelman WN, McCredie K, Trujillo JM, Broxmeyer HE, Henney C, Gutterman JU: Effects of recombinant human granulocyte-macrophage colony-stimulating factor in patients with myelodysplastic syndrome. N Engl J Med 1987;317:1545–1552.
118 Negrin RS, Haeuber DH, Nagler A, Kobayashi Y, et al: Maintenance treatment of patients with myelodysplastic syndromes using G-CSF. Blood 1990;76:36–43.
119 Ganser A, Ottmann OG, Schulz G, Hoelzer D: Recombinant human GM-CSF and low-dose cytosine arabinoside in pa-

tients with myelodysplastic syndrome. A pilot study. Onkologie 1989;12:13–15.
120 Storb R, Epstien R, Thomas E, et al: Marrow repopulating ability of peripheral blood cells compared to thoracic duct cells. Blood 1968;32:662–667.
121 Richman CM, Weiner RS, Yankee RA: Increase in circulating stem cells following chemotherapy in man. Blood 1976;47: 1031–1039.
122 Socinski MA, Cannistra SA, Elias A, Antman KH, Schnipper L, Griffin JD: Granulocyte-macrophage colony stimulating factor expands the circulating hematopoietic progenitor cell compartment in man. Lancet 1988;i:1194–1198.
123 Gianni AM, Siena S, Bregni M, Tarella C, et al: Granulocyte-macrophage colony-stimulating factor to harvest circulating hematopoietic stem cells for autotransplantation. Lancet 1989;i:580–584.
124 Gianni AM, Siena S, Bregni M, Tarella C, et al: Circulation of $CD34^+$ hematopoietic stem cells in the peripheral blood of high-dose cyclophosphamide-treated patients: Enhancement by intravenous rhGM-CSF. Blood 1989;74:1905–1914.
125 Kessinger A, Armitage JO, Smith DM, Landmark JD, Bierman PJ, Weisenburger DD: High-dose therapy and autologous peripheral blood stem cell transplantation for patients with lymphoma. Blood 1989;74:1260–1265.
126 Neidhart JA, Kohler W, Stidley C, Mangalik A, Plauche A, et al: Phase I study of repeated cycles of high-dose cyclophosphamide, etoposide, and cisplatin administered without bone marrow transplantation. J Clin Oncol 1990;8:1728–1738.
127 Nemunaitis J, Meyers JD, Buckner CD, Bianco JC, et al: Phase I/II trial of rhM-CSF in patients with invasive fungal infection (abstract No 625). Blood 1990;76(suppl 1):159a.
128 Pluda JM, Yarchoan R, Smith PD, Mc Atee N, Shay LE, et al: Subcutaneous recombinant GM-CSF used as a single agent and in an alternating regimen with azidothymidine in leukopenic patients with severe human immunodeficiency virus infection. Blood 1990;76:463–472.
129 Groopman JE: Status of colony-stimulating factors in cancer and AIDS. Semin Oncol 1990;17:31–37.
130 Andreesen R, Brugger W, Gadd S, Löhr GW, Atkins RC: Activation of human monocyte-derived macrophages cultured on Teflon. Response to interferon-gamma during terminal maturation in vitro. Immunobiology 1988;177:186–198.
131 Adams DO, Hall T, Steplewksi Z, et al: Tumor undergoing rejection induced by monoclonal antibodies of the IgG2a isotype contain increased numbers of macrophages and activated to a distinctive form of antibody dependent cytolysis. Proc Natl Acad Sci USA 1984;81:3506–3510.
132 Munn DH, Garnick MB, Cheung NK: Effects of parenteral recombinant human macrophage colony-stimulating factor on monocyte number, phenotype, and antitumor cytotoxicity in nonhuman primates. Blood 1990;75:2042–2048.
133 Zhou YQ, Stanley ER, Steven SC, Hatzfeld JA, et al: Interleukin-3 and interleukin-1 alpha allow earlier bone marrow progenitors to respond to human CSF-1. Blood 1988;72: 1870–1874.
134 Ikebuchi K, Wong CC, Clark SC, Ihle JN, Hirai W, Ogawa M: Interleukin-6 enhancement of interleukin-3 dependent proliferation of multipotential hemopoietic progenitors. PNAS 1987;84:9035–9039.
135 Futami H, Jansen R, Irino S, Keller J, Longo DL, Oppenheim JJ, Ruscetti FW, Wiltrout RH: Chemoprotective effects of rhIL-1a in normal and tumor-bearing mice (abstract). Proc AACR 1990;31:294.
136 Asano S, Okano A, Ozawa K, Nakahata T, Ishibashi T, et al: In vivo effects of rhIL-6 in primates: stimulated production of platelets. Blood 1990;75:1602–1605.
137 Zeidler C, Souza L, Welte K: In vivo effects of interleukin-6 on hematopoiesis in primates. Blood 1989;74:154a.
138 Zeidler C, Kanz L, Pietsch T, Boone T, Samal B, Welte K: Leukemia inhibitory factor (LIF) induces thrombocytosis in primates. Blood 1990;76(suppl 1):174a.
139 Kanz L, Kostielniak E, Welte K: Colony-stimulating activity unique for the megakaryocytic hemopoietic cell lineage, present in the plasma of a patient with the syndrome of thrombocytopenia with absent radii (TAR). Blood 1989;74:248a.
140 Zsebo KM, Wypych J, McNiece IK, Lu HS, Smith KA, Karkare SB, et al: Identification, purification, and biological characterization of hematopoietic stem cell factor from buffalo rat liver-conditioned medium. Cell 1990;63:195–201.
141 Martin FH, Suggs SV, Langley KW; Lu HS, Ting J, et al: Primary structure and functional expression of rat and human stem cell factor DNAs. Cell 1990;63:203–211.
142 Andrews RG, Bartelmez SH, Egrie J, Bernstein ID, Zsebo K: Recombinant human stem cell factor stimulates in vitro and in vivo hematopoiesis in baboons. Blood 1990;76(suppl 1): 130a.

Roland Mertelsmann, MD, PhD
Department of Hematology and Oncology
University of Freiburg Medical Center
Hugstetter Strasse 55
D-W-7800 Freiburg (FRG)

Acta Haematol 1991;86:148–154

0001–5792/91/0863–0148 $ 2.75/0

The Role of Interleukin-1 in Hematopoiesis

W.E. Fibbe, R. Willemze

Department of Hematology, University Medical Center Leiden, The Netherlands

Key Words. Colony-stimulating factor · Cytokines · Gene expression · Hematopoiesis · Hematopoietic growth factor · Myelosuppression

Abstract. The polypeptide interleukin 1 (IL-1) is the primary mediator of the acute-phase response and is responsible for many changes that are associated with the onset of infection. It induces fever and has profound endocrinologic metabolic and hematologic effects. Two structurally related forms of IL-1 have been described, termed IL-1α and IL-1β. Both forms of IL-1 bind to a common receptor that is present on a variety of target cells. Recently, IL-1 has been recognized as a molecule that is important in the regulation of hematopoiesis. IL-1 induces the production of several different hematopoietic growth factors including granulocyte-macrophage, granulocyte and macrophage colony-stimulating factors and interleukin 6 by a variety of accessory cells. In addition, IL-1 acts synergistically with colony-stimulating factors in the proliferation of primitive hematopoietic progenitor cells. In vivo, the administration of IL-1 accelerates hematopoietic reconstitution after chemotherapy or radiation induced myelosuppression. In untreated animals, IL-1 may induce a shift of hematopoietic progenitor cells into the peripheral blood, and these cells may be used to repopulate the bone marrow of lethally irradiated recipients. These studies suggest that IL-1 may be used as a therapeutic agent to accelerate bone marrow recovery after myelosuppression.

Introduction

Interleukin-1 (IL-1) is a pleiotropic cytokine with multiple biologic activities. It is considered to be the primary mediator of the acute phase response and is responsible for many of the changes associated with infection. There are two structurally related IL-1 molecules named IL-1α and IL-1β. The genes for these molecules are both located on chromosome 2. Both forms of IL-1 bind to a single class of receptors present on a variety of cell types that respond to IL-1 in vitro, i.e. lymphocytes, fibroblasts, endothelial cells and many other cell types. Cells of the mononuclear phagocytic lineage are considered the main source of IL-1 production. Both forms of IL-1 are translated as precursor proteins of approximately 31 kD. Whereas the precursor form of IL-1β requires conversion into its mature form of 17 kD to exert biologic activity, the IL-1α precursor protein is able to bind to the receptor and to exert bioactivity.

The involvement of IL-1 in the regulation of hematopoiesis has been reported in early studies using a partially purified IL-1 molecule that was designated as leukocytic endogenous mediator [1, 2]. Since then, numerous studies using purified and recombinant IL-1 molecules have further substantiated the role of IL-1 in hematopoiesis. In the present review, the effects on normal and leukemic hematopoietic cells will be discussed.

Induction of Growth Factors

In cultures of human bone marrow cells, IL-1 induces a dose-dependent stimulatory effect on colony formation [3]. This effect appears to be indirect and is mediated by accessory cells present in the marrow suspensions. Depletion of mononuclear phagocytes almost entirely abrogates the stimulatory activities of IL-1, whereas media conditioned by purified mononuclear phagocytes in the presence of IL-1 contain a colony-stimulating activity (CSA).

These results indicate that IL-1 induces the production of colony-stimulating factors (CSF) by mononuclear phagocytes. A variety of other cell populations of accessory cells can be induced by IL-1 to produce stimulating activities, i.e. human fibroblasts [4, 5], bone marrow stromal cells [6] or endothelial cells [7–9] produce CSA for myeloid (CFU-GM), erythroid (BFU-E) and multipotent (CFU-GEMM) progenitor cells. These activities have been identified as granulocyte (G-CSF) and granulocyte-macrophage (GM-CSF), both at a protein and mRNA level [10–15]. Studies on the production of macrophage CSF (M-CSF) by fibroblasts have yielded contradictory results. Some groups have reported constitutive production of M-CSF by both fibroblasts and endothelial cells [9–11], whereas others have found IL-1-inducible production of M-CSF [12]. Recent studies indicate that these apparently contradictory results may be explained by the culture conditions used to study M-CSF production [15]. Fibroblasts cultured under serum-limiting conditions become quiescent and growth arrested. These cells do not incorporate ^{3}H-thymidine, exhibit little expression of M-CSF, as demonstrated by Northern blot analysis and produce only small amounts of M-CSF protein. Following addition of fetal bovine serum or various fibroblast growth-promoting factors, proliferation of fibroblasts and M-CSF transcription can be reinduced. Similarly, IL-1 induces an increase in M-CSF expression, not only in quiescent fibroblasts but also in proliferating fibroblasts cultured in the presence of serum. The increase in M-CSF production induced by IL-1 appears to be controlled at the level of transcription. This contrasts to the IL-1-induced production of GM-CSF that has been found to be controlled by stabilization of mRNA [16].

In long-term bone marrow cultures, addition of IL-1 results in high concentrations of CSA in the supernatant [17]. The presence of immunoreactive G-CSF, M-CSF and GM-CSF has been demonstrated in the supernatants. Similar results have been reported for human bone-marrow-derived fibroblastoid stromal cells after stimulation by IL-1 [18, 19]. Finally, activated T lymphocytes can be induced by IL-1 to produce GM-CSF [20] and presumably also IL-3.

Effect of IL-1 on Hematopoietic Progenitor Cells

The survival of hematopoietic progenitor cells (HPC) in vitro requires the presence of hematopoietic growth factors. In the absence of growth factors and when cultured under conditions that preclude endogenous production of growth factors, HPC die within several days [21]. The in vitro survival of both murine [22] and human [23] HPC is significantly enhanced by IL-1. In the absence of CSF, i.e. on bone marrow cell suspensions that have been depleted of accessory cells, this effect of IL-1 was maintained, suggesting that it was not mediated by intermediate production of CSF. Furthermore, the survival of CFU-GM and BFU-E, in cultures of low-density bone marrow cells, can be decreased by addition of an anti-IL-1 antiserum, indicating that endogenous production of IL-1 contributes to the in vitro survival of these cells. Thus, IL-1 enhances the survival of progenitor cells in the absence of CSF by mechanisms that have not been identified yet.

Several synergistic activities of IL-1 have been reported on the growth of HPC. On relatively mature progenitor cells, IL-1 and GM-CSF exhibited a synergistic effect on the growth of CFU-GM [24, 25]. This effect was preserved in cultures of monocyte- and T-lymphocyte-depleted cells, but was not present anymore when CD34-enriched marrow suspensions were used [24]. These results indicated that the synergistic effect was mediated by an intermediate factor produced in response to IL-1. Neutralization studies showed that the production of G-CSF by residual accessory cells was responsible for the synergistic effect. On relatively immature progenitor cells, other synergistic effects have been reported. A synergistic factor obtained from media conditioned by 5637 bladder carcinoma cells, designated as hemopoietin 1, has been identified by Jubinski, Stanley and Bartelmez [26–28]. This factor was subsequently identified as IL-1, and in the presence of M-CSF, it induced the growth of large colonies that were called high-proliferative potential colony-forming cells. These colonies were derived from mouse bone marrow cells, obtained from animals that were pretreated with 5-fluorouracil and thus depleted of relatively mature HPC and enriched for resting progenitor cells. Addition of single lineage CSF induced no colony growth on these cell suspensions. Similarly, IL-1 alone had no direct colony-stimulatory effect, but the combination of IL-1 and M-CSF or even more the combination of IL-1,

M-CSF and interleukin 3 (IL-3) induced the formation of giant colonies [29]. Upon replating, secondary colonies were formed, suggesting the involvement of primitive HPC.

Interleukin 6 (IL-6) represents another factor that acts synergistically with IL-3 on the poliferation of immature murine HPC, derived from 5-fluorouracil-pretreated mice [30, 31]. Since the production of IL-6 is induced by IL-1 [32], the possibility was considered that the synergistic effect of IL-1 was due to intermediate production of IL-6. On human HPC that have been purified with anti-CD34 monoclonal antibodies, a synergistic effect of the combination of IL-3 and IL-6 has been found on the growth of multilineage blast cell colonies [33]. In this system, IL-1 did not show the synergistic activities with IL-3. These results were interpreted to imply that IL-1 has no direct synergistic effect on early stem cells, and that intermediate production of IL-6 is responsible for the synergistic activities by shortening the G0 period of the cell cycle and by inducing expression of receptors for other growth factors.

Effect of IL-1 on Leukemic Cells

CSF may play a role in the growth of malignant hematopoietic cells obtained from patients with acute myelogenous leukemia (AML). These cells may exhibit spontaneous growth due to the constitutive production of CSF in an autocrine fashion. IL-1 has also been suggested as a growth-promoting molecule for AML blasts. These cells may produce IL-1, and anti-IL-1 antibodies may abrogate the spontaneous proliferation of these cells [34, 35]. Rambaldi et al. [36] have used the recombinant IL-1 receptor-antagonist protein to study the role of IL-1 on 'spontaneous' growth of AML cells. They also found a significant inhibition in the majority of the cases studied, indicating that autocrine IL-1 production contributed to the spontaneous proliferation. These studies indicate that IL-1 may act as a direct or indirect autocrine growth factor for AML cells. In patients with chronic lymphocytic leukemia or multiple myeloma [37, 38], IL-1 has been found to accelerate the autocrine growth of malignant cells, through the production of IL-6. Acute lymphoblastic leukemia cell lines may also be responsive to IL-1, and addition of IL-1 alone or in combination with other factors may induce growth of these cells [39–41], without concurrent differentiation.

In vivo Hematopoietic Effect of IL-1

Because IL-1 has multiple hematopoietic effects by inducing production of hematopoietic growth factors and by acting synergistically with these factors on various populations of primitive or committed progenitor cells, it may be a potential candidate for stimulating hematopoiesis in vivo. In rabbits or mice, IL-1 injection results in a dose-dependent granulocytosis [42]. This increase in neutrophils is accompanied by a significant increase in the number of circulating HPC. For instance, a mean 20-fold increase in the number of CFU-GM can be reached at 4–8 h after a single intraperitoneal injection of IL-1 in mice [43]. Also, plasma levels of CSA were significantly higher in animals treated with IL-1α [44].

The effects of IL-1 treatment on bone marrow recovery have been studied in mice treated with sublethal doses of cyclophosphamide or irradiation [45–47]. Treatment with IL-1 accelerated the recovery of neutrophils, accompanied by an increased number of CFU-GM in the bone marrow. The injection of IL-1 to animals that were pretreated with 5-fluorouracil resulted in accelerated marrow reconstitution. Injection with G-CSF was equally effective as IL-1, whereas a combination of IL-1 and G-CSF acted synergistically [48]. We have found that a single dose of IL-1 administered to mice with cyclophosphamide-induced neutropenia accelerated neutrophil recovery in mice [49]. In these animals, an increased bone marrow cellularity was found in IL-1-treated animals. Johnson et al. [50] observed an increase in the number of progenitor cells in the bone marrow and spleen, 2 days after injection of IL-1. The increase included the number of myeloid (CFU-GM) and early erythroid (BFU-E) progenitor cells, whereas a suppresive effect on the mature erythroid progenitor cells (CFU-E) was found. The latter effect could be abrogated by simultaneous administration of erythropoietin.

Recent evidence suggest that IL-1 not only affects the reconstitution of neutrophils, but also of platelets. The first notion came from in vivo studies in primates where an increase in the number of platelets was found after IL-1 injection [51]. Recently, several groups have found that IL-6 potentiates in vitro megakaryocytopoiesis in mice [52–54] and humans [55, 56]. In vivo, IL-6 has been found to be a potent stimulator on thrombopoiesis in untreated mice [57, 58] and primates [59]. Similarly, repeated injections of IL-1β to mice induced thrombocytosis [60]. Since these animals had high levels of IL-6 in the serum, it is likely that the thrombocytosis was mediated by intermediate production of IL-6.

Radioprotection

Mice pretreated with IL-1 followed by the administration of sublethal dose of irradiation may be rescued from the otherwise lethal effect of irradiation on the bone marrow [61–64]. A single dose of 200 ng of IL-1α was radioprotective when administered 20 or 4 h before irradiation [64]. Administration of IL-1 at 48 h before radiation, however, was completely ineffective in mediating radioprotection. The basis for these protective effects remains largely unknown. It may reflect the ability of IL-1 to induce hematopoietic growth factors that accelerate hematopoietic recovery, or to induce other unknown factors which have direct protective effects on progenitor cells. Another hypothesis is that the protective mechanism may be cell-cycle-specific in that cells in the late S phase of the cycle are relatively resistant to radiation damage [65].

Preliminary Experience in Humans

In view of its multiple hematopoietic effects, it may be possible that deficiency of IL-1 contributes to the development of bone marrow failure. In contrast to the numerous studies on the role of IL-1 in the 'inducible' hematopoiesis, it is still unknown whether IL-1 has a physiologic role in steady-state hematopoiesis. In patients with aplastic anemia, decreased IL-1 production by monocytes has been found [66, 67], although the role in the pathogenesis of this disorder is as yet difficult to establish. Conversely, there are indications that the prolonged endogenous production of IL-1 is associated with the development of anemia of chronic disease. In accordance, terminal erythroid differentiation is suppressed by IL-1 [50].

The preliminary clinical experience with IL-1 has focussed on its hematopoietic effects and on its possible antitumor activity. Recombinant human IL-1β has been administered as 30-min infusions for 5 days to patients with metastatic malignant disorders [68]. The main side effects included an increase in heart rate, a decrease in blood pressure, induction of monophasic fever and chills, headache and local erythema at the site of injection. IL-1 administration induced a rise in neutrophil counts in all patients between 4 and 8 h after initiating treatment, suggesting that this effect was due to a shift from the bone marrow to the peripheral blood. Platelet counts showed a rise of 50% occurring 6 days after beginning the treatment and lasting for 24 days after treatment.

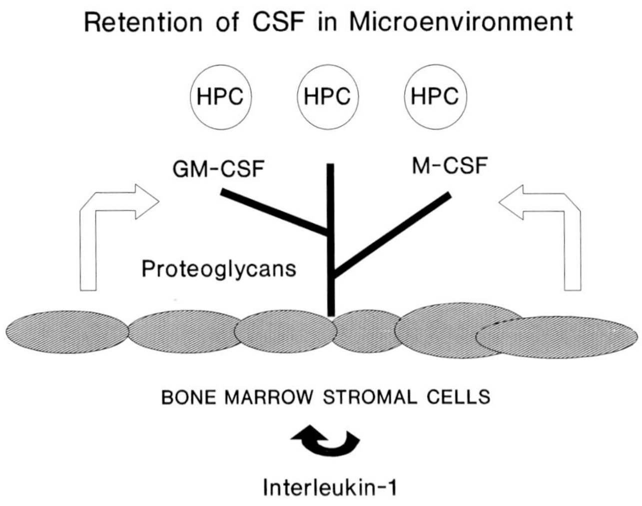

Fig. 1. IL-1 may induce the production of CSF in the bone marrow stroma in a paracrine fashion. These CSF are retained in the bone marrow microenvironment by binding to proteoglycans and may be presented to HPC.

Therefore, this effect may result from stimulated megakaryopoiesis in the bone marrow. However, no bone marrow studies have been performed in these patients. Although plasma levels of GM-CSF, IL-3 or IL-6 were not increased in these patients, it remains possible that the effects on platelet counts are mediated by IL-6 production, occurring at concentrations that were below the detection limit of the assays used. It is also possible that IL-1 induces the production of these cytokines in the bone marrow microenvironment directly through a paracrine mechanism, without inducing circulating levels of these cytokines (fig. 1).

A myeloprotective effect of IL-1 has been observed in patients with metastatic colorectal cancer treated with IL-1β in a phase I/II trial [69–71]. These preliminary studies suggest that IL-1 may be used to accelerate the recovery of neutrophils and platelets in patients receiving chemotherapy. Possible advantages of

Table 1. Potential advantages of IL-1 in vivo treatment

Effect on neutrophils and platelets
Induction of multiple CSF
Induction of CSF in bone marrow microenvironment
Synergy with CSF
Immature target HPC
Effective short duration of treatment

IL-1 treatment include the induction of growth factors in the bone marrow microenvironment itself, a synergistic effect between IL-1-induced CSF and IL-1, and its effect on platelet counts (table 1). It is important to note that most effects of IL-1 are observed after a single injection. Animal studies even suggest that prolonged administration of IL-1 may be counterproductive by the induction of suppressive molecules like tumor necrosis factor [72]. Since IL-1 acts on a primitive hematopoietic target cell, it may also be a potential candidate for combination or sequential treatment with CSF.

In conclusion, the preliminary evidence with IL-1 as a therapeutic agent suggests that short-term and low-dose treatment may be beneficial by augmenting host-defense systems. Carefully designed trials are required to define the ultimate role of this molecule in the treatment of hematologic disorders.

Acknowledgement

We thank Miss D. van Ruiten for typing this manuscript.

References

1 Kampschmidt RF, Upchurch HF: Possible involvement of leukocytic endogenous mediator in granulopoiesis. Proc Soc Exp Biol Med 1977;155:89–93.
2 Willemze R, Walker RI, Herion JC, Palmer JG: Marrow culture in diffusion chambers in rabbits. III. Effect of endotoxin and leukocyte products on cell production. Am J Hematol 1979;7:33–43.
3 Fibbe WE, Van Damme J, Billiau A, Voogt PJ, Duinkerken N, Kluck PMC, Falkenburg JHF: Interleukin-1 (22-K factor) induces release of granulocyte-macrophage colony-stimulating activity from human mononuclear phagocytes. Blood 1986;68:1316–1321.
4 Zucali JR, Dinarello CA, Oblon DJ, Gross MA, Anderson L, Weiner RS: Interleukin 1 stimulates fibroblasts to produce granulocyte-macrophage colony-stimulating activity and prostaglandin E_2. J Clin Invest 1986;77:1857–1863.
5 Zucali JR, Broxmeyer HE, Dinarello CA, Gross MA, Weiner RS: Regulation of early human hematopoietic (BFU-E and CFU-GEMM) progenitor cells in vitro by interleukin 1-induced fibroblast-conditioned medium. Blood 1987;69:33–37.
6 Lovhaug D, Pelus LM, Nordlie EM, Boyum A, Moore MAS: Monocyte-conditioned medium and interleukin 1 induce granulocyte-macrophage colony-stimulating factor production in the adherent cell layer of murine bone marrow cultures. Exp Hematol 1986;14:1037–1042.
7 Bagby GC Jr, Dinarello CA, Wallace P, Wagner C, Hefeneider S, McCall E: Interleukin 1 stimulates granulocyte-macrophage colony-stimulating activity release by vascular endothelial cells. J Clin Invest 1986;78:1316–1323.
8 Segal GM, McCall E, Stueve T, Bagby GC Jr: Interleukin 1 stimulates endothelial cells to release multlineage human colony-stimulating activity. J Immunol 1987;6:1772–1778.
9 Segal GM, McCall E, Stueve T, Bagby GC: Interleukin 1 stimulates endothelial cells to release multilineage human colony-stimulating activity. J Immunol 1987;138:1772–1778.
10 Broudy VC, Kaushansky K, Harlan JM, Adamson JW: Interleukin 1 stimulates human endothelial cells to produce granulocyte-macrophage colony-stimulating factor and granulocyte colony-stimulating factor. J Immunol 1987;139:464–468.
11 Kaushansky K, Lin N, Adamson JW: Interleukin 1 stimulates fibroblasts to synthesize granulocyte-macrophage and granulocyte colony-stimulating factors. J Clin Invest 1988;81:92–97.
12 Fibbe WE, Van Damme J, Billiau A, Duinkerken N, Lurvink E, Ralph P, Altrock BW, Kaushansky K, Willemze R, Falkenburg JHF: Human fibroblasts produce granulocyte-CSF, macrophage-CSF and granulocyte-macrophage-CSF following stimulation by interleukin-1 and poly(rI).poly(rC). Blood 1988;72:860–866.
13 Fibbe WE, Daha MR, Hiemstra PS, Duinkerken N, Nurvink E, Ralph PR, Altrock BW, Kaushansky K, Willemze R, Falkenburg JHF: Interleukin-1 and poly(rI).poly(rC) induce production of granulocyte CSF, macrophage CSF, and granulocyte-macrophage CSF by human endothelial cells. Exp Hematol 1989;17:229–234.
14 Sieff CA, Schickwann F, Faller DV: Interleukin 1 induces cultured human endothelial cell production of granulocyte-macrophage colony-stimulating factor. J Clin Invest 1987;79:48–51.
15 Falkenburg JHF, Harrington MA, Walsh WK, Daub R, Broxmeyer HE: Regulation of gene-expression and release of macrophage colony-stimulating factor in quiescent and proliferating fibroblasts: Effects of serum, fibroblast growth-promoting factors and interleukin-1. Submitted for publication.
16 Bagby GC, Shaw G, Brown MA, Damm D, Hefeneider S, Heinrich M, Band L, Segal GM: IL-1 induces GM-CSF gene expression by activating ribonuclease inhibitors (abstract). Blood 1988;72(suppl 1):109a.
17 Fibbe WE, Van Damme J, Billiau A, Goselink HM, Voogt PJ, van Eeden G, Ralph P, Altrock BW, Falkenburg JHF: Interleukin-1 induces human marrow stromal cells in long-term culture to produce granulocyte colony-stimulating factor and macrophage colony-stimulating factor. Blood 1988;71:430–435.
18 Rennick D, Yang G, Gemmell L, Lee F: Control of hemopoiesis by a bone marrow stromal cell clone: Lipopolysaccharide- and interleukin-1-inducible production of colony-stimulating factors. Blood 1987;69:682–691.

19 Broudy VC, Zuckerman KS, Jetmalani S, Fitchen JH, Bagby GC Jr: Monocytes stimulate fibroblastoid bone marrow stromal cells to produce multilineage hematopoietic growth factors. Blood 1986;68:530–534.
20 Herrmann F, Oster W, Meuer CS, Lindenmann A, Mertelsmann RH: Interleukin 1 stimulates T lymphocytes to produce granulocyte-monocyte colony-stimulating factor. J Clin Invest 1988;81:1415–1418.
21 Metcalf D, Merchav S: Effects of GM-CSF deprivation on precursors of granulocytes and macrophages. J Cell Physiol 1982; 112:411–418.
22 Williams DE, Broxmeyer HE: Interleukin-1 alpha enhances the in-vitro survival of purified murine granulocyte-macrophage progenitor cells in the absence of colony-stimulating factors. Blood 1988;72:1608–1615.
23 Hangoc G, Williams DE, Falkenburg JHF, Broxmeyer HE: Influence of IL-1α and IL-1β on the survival of human bone marrow cells responding to haematopoietic colony-stimulating factors. J Immunol 1989;142:4329–4334.
24 Schaafsma MR, Falkenburg JHF, Duinkerken N, Van Damme J, Altrock BW, Willemze R, Fibbe WE: Interleukin-1 synergizes with granulocyte-macrophage colony-stimulating factor on granulocytic colony formation by intermediate production of granulocyte colony-stimulating factor. Blood 1989;74:2398–2404.
25 Hoang T, Haman A, Goncalves O, Letendre F, Mathieu M, Wong GC, Clark SC: Interleukin-1 enhances growth factor-dependent proliferation of the clonogenic cells in acute myeloblastic leukemia and of normal human primitive hemopoietic precusors. J Exp Med 1988;168:463–474.
26 Jubinsky PT, Stanley ER: Purification of hemopoietin-1: A multilineage hemopoietic growth factor. Proc Natl Acad Sci USA 1985;82:2764–2768.
27 Stanley ER, Bartocci A, Patinkin D, Rosendaal M, Bradley TR: Regulation of very primitive, multipotent, hemopoietic cells by hemopoietin-1. Cell 1987;45:667–674.
28 Bartelmez SH, Stanley ER: Synergism between hemopoietic growth factors (HFG's) detected by their effects on cells bearing receptors for a lineage specific HGF: Assay of hemopoietin-1. J Cell Physiol 1985;122:370–378.
29 Bartelmez SH, Bradley TR, Bertoncello I, Mochizuki DY, Tushinski RJ, Stanley ER, Hapel AJ, Young IG, Kregler AB, Hodgson GS: Interleukin 1 plus interleukin 3 plus colony-stimulating factor 1 are essential for clonal proliferation of primitive myeloid bone marrow cells. Exp Hematol 1989;17:240–245.
30 Ikebuchi K, Wong GG, Clark SC, Ihle JN, Hiria Y, Ogawa M: Interleukin 6 enhancement of interleukin 3-dependent proliferation of multipotential hemopoietic progenitors. Proc Natl Acad Sci USA 1987;84:9035–9039.
31 Ikebuchi K, Ihle JN, Hirai Y, Wong GG, Clark SC, Ogawa M: Synergistic factors for stem cell proliferation: Further studies of the target stem cells and the mechanism of stimulation by interleukin-1, interleukin-6, and granulocyte colony-stimulating factor. Blood 1988;72:2007–2014.
32 Van Damme J, Cayphas S, Opdenakker G, Billia A, Van Snick J: Interleukin 1 and poly(rI).poly(rC) induce production by a hybridoma growth factor by human fibroblasts. Eur J Immunol 1987;17:1–7.
33 Leary AG, Ikebuchi K, Hirai Y, Wong GG, Yng Y, Clark SC, Ogawa M: Synergism between interleukin-6 and interleukin-3 in supporting proliferation of human hematopoietic stem cells: Comparison with interleukin-1α. Blood 1988;71:1759–1763.
34 Cozzolino F, Rubartelli A, Aldinucci D et al: Interleukin-1 as an autocrine growth factor for acute myeloid leukemia cells. Proc Natl Acad Sci USA 1989;86:2369–2373.
35 Griffin JD, Rambaldi A, Vellenga E, Young DC, Octaporicz D, Cannistra SA: Secretion of interleukin-1 by acute myeloblastic leukemia cells in vitro induces endothelial cells to secrete colony stimulating factors. Blood 1987;70:1218–1221.
36 Rambaldi A, Torcia M, Bettoni S, Vannier E, Barbui T, Dinarello CA, Cozzolino F: Modulation of cell proliferation and cytokine production in acute myeloblastic leukemia by recombinant IL-1 receptor antagonist and lack of its expression by leukemic cells (abstract). Blood 1990;76(suppl 1):114a.
37 Kawano M, Tanaka H, Ishikawa H et al: Interleukin-1 accelerates autocrine growth of myeloma cells through interleukin-6 in human myeloma. Blood 1989;73:2145–2148.
38 Biondi A, Rossi V, Bassan R et al: Constitutive expression of the interleukin-6 gene in chronic lymphocytic leukemia. Blood 1989;73:1270–1284.
39 Uchun FM, Myers DE, Fauci AS, Chandan-Langlie M, Ambrus JL: Leukemic B-cell precursors constitutively express functional receptor for human interleukin-1. Blood 1989;74: 761–776.
40 Uckun FM, Ledbetter JA: Immunobiologic differences between normal and leukemic human B-cell precursors. Proc Natl Acad Sci USA 1988;85:8603–8607.
41 Uckun FM, Gesner TG, Song CW, Myers DE, Mufson A: Leukemic B-cell precursors express functional receptors for human interleukin-3. Blood 1989;73:533–542.
42 Van Damme J, Opdenakker G, De Ley M, Heremans H, Billiau A: Pyrogenic and haematological effects of the interferon-inducing 22K factor (interleukin-1) from human leukocytes. Clin Exp Immunol 1986;66:303–311.
43 Fibbe WE, Hamilton MS, Laterveer LL, Kibbelaar RE, Falkenburg JHF, Visser JWM, Willemze R: Sustained engraftment of mice transplanted with peripheral blood-derived interleukin-1 primed stem cells. J Immunol (in press).
44 Vogel SN, Douches SD, Kaufman EN, Neta R: Induction of colony-stimulating factor in vivo by recombinant interleukin-1α and recombinant tumor necrosis factor-α. J Immunol 1987;128:2143–2148.
45 Gallicchio VS: Accelerated recovery of hematopoiesis following sub-lethal whole body irradiation with recombinant murine interleukin-1 (IL-1). J Leukocyte Biol 1988;43:211–215.
46 Stork L, Barczuk L, Kissinger M, Robinson W: Interleukin-1 accelerates murine granulocyte recovery following treatment with cyclophosphamide. Blood 1989;73:938–944.
47 Benjamin WR, Tare NS, Hayes TJ, Becker JM, Anderson TD: Regulation of hemopoiesis in myelosuppressed mice by human recombinant IL-1α. J Immunol 1989;142:792–799.
48 Moore MAS, Waren DJ: Synergy of interleukin-1 and granulocyte colony stimulating factor: In vivo stimulation of stem-cell recovery and hematopoietic regeneration following 5-fluorouracil treatment of mice. Proc Natl Acad Sci USA 1987;84: 7134–7138.
49 Fibbe WE, van der Meer JWM, Falkenburg JHF, Hamilton MS, Kluin PM, Dinarello CA: A single low dose of human recombinant interleukin-1 accelerates the recovery of neutro-

phils in mice with cyclophosphamide-induced neutropenia. Exp Hematol 1989;17:805–808.
50 Johnson CS, Keckler DJ, Topper MI, Braunschweiger PG, Furmanski P: In vivo hematopoietic effects of recombinant interleukin-1α in mice: Stimulation of granulocytic, monocytic, megakaryocytic, and early erythroid progenitors, suppression of late-stage erythropoiesis and reversal of erythroid suppression with erythropoietin. Blood 1989;73:678–683.
51 Monroy RL, Skelly RR, Davis TA, Benjamin W, Lomedico P, Dinarello CA, Donahue RE, MacVittie TJ: Effect of interleukin-1 on the recovery of primates after radiation and autologous bone marrow transplantation (abstract). Blood 1987; 70:321a.
52 Ishibashi T, Kimura H, Uchida T, Kariyone S, Friese P, Burstein SA: Human interleukin 6 as a direct promotor of maturation of megakaryocytes in vitro. Proc Natl Acad Sci USA 1989;86:5953–5957.
53 Lotem J, Shabo Y, Sachs L: Regulation of megakaryocyte development of interleukin-6. Blood 1989;74:1545–1551.
54 McGrath HE, McNiece IK, Clark S, Gillis S, Queseberry PJ: Interleukin-6 stimulation of murine megakaryocyte colony formation (abstract). Clin Res 1989;37:549a.
55 Bruno E, Hoffman R: Effect of interleukin 6 on in vitro human megakaryocytopoiesis: Its interaction with other cytokines. Exp Hematol 1989;17:1038–1043.
56 Kimura H, Ishibashi T, Uchida T, Maruyama Y, Friese P, Burstein SA: Interleukin 6 is a differentiation factor for human megakaryocytes in vitro. Eur J Immunol 1990;20:1927–1931.
57 Ishibashi T, Kimura H, Shikama Y, Uchida T, Kariyone S, Hirano T, Kishimoto T, Takatsuki F, Akiyama Y: Interleukin-6 is a potent thrombopoietic factor in vivo in mice. Blood 1989; 74:1241–1244.
58 Hill RJ, Warren MK, Levin J: Stimulation of thrombopoiesis in mice by human recombinant Interleukin 6. J Clin Invest 1990; 85:1242–1247.
59 Asano S, Ozawa K, Nakahata T, Ishibashi T, Koike K, Kimura H, Tanioka Y, Shibuya A, Hirano T, Kishimoto T, Takaku F, Akiyama Y: In vivo effects of recombinant human interleukin-6 in primates: Stimulated production of platelets. Blood 1990;75:1602–1605.
60 Kimura H, Ishibashi T, Shikama Y, Okano A, Akiyama Y, Uchida T, Maruyama Y: Interleukin-1β (IL-1β) induces thrombocytosis in mice: Possible implification of IL-6. Blood 1990; 76:2493–2500.
61 Behling NM: The radioprotective effect of bacterial endotoxin; in Nowotny A (ed): Beneficial Effects of Endotoxins. New York, Plenum Publishing Corp, 1983, p 127.
62 Neta R, Vogel SN, Oppenheim JJ, Douches SD: Cytokines in radioprotection. Comparison of the radioprotective effects of IL-1 to IL-2, GM-CSF and IFNγ. Lymphokine Res 1986; 5(suppl 1);105–110.
63 Neta R, Douches S, Oppenheim JJ: Interleukin 1 is a radioprotector. J Immunol 1986;136:2483–2485.
64 Neta R, Oppenheim JJ, Douches SD, Giclas PC, Imbra RJ, Karin M: Radioprotection with interleukin-1: Comparison with other cytokines. Prog Immunol 1986;IV:900–908.
65 Talmadge JE, Herbermann RB, Chirigos MA et al: Hyporesponsiveness to augmentation of murine natural killer cell activity in different anatomical compartments by multiple injections of various immunomodulators including recombinant interferons and interleukin-2. J Immunol 1985;135:2483.
66 Gascon P, Scala G: Decreased Interleukin-1 production in aplastic anemia. Am J Med 1988;85:668–674.
67 Nakao S, Matushima K, Young N: Decreased interleukin-1 production in aplastic anemia. Br J Haematol 1989;71:431–436.
68 Tewari A, Buhles WC, Starnes HF: Preliminary report: Effects of interleukin-1 on platelet counts. Lancet 1990;336:712–714.
69 Crown J, Kemeny N, Jakubowski A et al: Phase I-II trial of recombinant human interleukin-1B (IL-1) in patients with metastatic colorectal cancer receiving 5-fluorouracil (abstract). Blood 1989;74(suppl 1):15.
70 Crown J, Gabrilove J, Kemeny N et al: Phase I-I trial of human recombinant interleukin-1B (IL-1) in patients with metastatic colorectal cancer (MCC) receiving myelosuppressive doses of 5-fluorouracil (5-FU) (abstract). Proc Am Soc Clin Oncol 1990;90:183.
71 Smith J II, Urba W, Steis R et al: Interleukin-1 alpha: Results of a phase I toxicity and immunomodulatory trial (abstract). Proc Am Soc Clin Oncol 1990;9:187.
72 Gasparetto C, Laver J, Abboud M, Gillio A, Smith C, O'Reilly RJ, Moore AS: Effect of interleukin-1 on hematopoietic progenitors: Evidence of stimulatory and inhibitory activities in a primate model. Blood 1989;74:547–550.

W.E. Fibbe, MD
Department of Hematology
University Medical Center
Building 1, 2C-R
PO Box 9600
NL–2300 RC Leiden (The Netherlands)

Acta Haematol 1991;86:155–161

0001–5792/91/0863–0155 $ 2.75/0

The Role of Haematopoietic Growth Factors in Bone Marrow Transplantation

E.E. Polli

Istituto di Scienze Mediche, Padiglione Granelli, Milano, Italia

Key Words. Bone marrow failure · Bone marrow transplantation · Haematopoietic growth factors · Peripheral stem cells transplantation

Abstract. Bone marrow transplantation (BMT) is being increasingly used for treating a large number of diseases. The recent availability of haematopoietic growth factors (HGFs) for therapeutic purposes has offered a powerful tool in order to overcome one of the most important BMT-related complications, namely severe myelosuppression. This article, besides an overview on the main results achieved with the clinical use of HGFs for haematopoietic reconstitution after BMT, also deals with some innovative applications of these molecules in BMT setting, as their use for peripheral stem cell transplantation and bone marrow failure after BMT.

Introduction

Human haematopoietic growth factors (HGFs) are a complex family of glycoproteins controlling the proliferation, differentiation and function of haematopoietic cell lineages. The development of recombinant DNA cloning technology has recently made possible the production of several HGFs on a scale large enough not only for extensive biological investigation but also for clinical trials aimed at assessing the therapeutic efficacy of these molecules. Bone marrow transplantation (BMT), an increasingly used treatment option for both solid tumours and haematologic malignancies, has been viewed as a promising setting for the clinical use of HGFs. The most obvious and so far most frequently investigated use of HGFs in BMT is to minimize the period of chemotherapy-induced cytopenia. Indeed, in BMT about half of the recorded deaths are associated with infective complications from either bacterial or fungal agents developing during severe myelosuppression. The administration of recombinant HGFs, by shortening the time for bone marrow repopulation after transplantation, would obviously lead to less morbidity and mortality due to cytopenias. Moreover, since also organ toxicity has been recently related to severity of neutropenia, methods for shortening the duration of myelosuppression might have an impact also on major organ toxicities [19]. In addition to the acceleration of haematopoietic reconstitution, there are other goals that might be achieved with the use of HGFs in BMT, as for instance improving the harvest of peripheral blood progenitor cells for autotransplantation, forcing leukaemic cells into the cell cycle before cytotoxic conditioning regimens, augmenting cellular response against infections and stimulating host anti-tumour reactivity.

This review will focus on the two so far most extensively studied HGFs in BMT, namely granulocyte colony-stimulating factor (G-CSF) and granulocyte-macrophage colony-stimulating factor (GM-CSF). The rationale for the clinical use of G-CSF and GM-CSF in BMT stems from the biological properties displayed by these factors both in vitro and in vivo.

The main effect of G-CSF on haematopoietic precursor cells both in vitro and in vivo is to promote the proliferation and differentiation of the granulocytic lineage [1, 2]. In in vitro systems, however, an activity on pluripotent precursor cells (CFU-GEMM) and early erythroid precursor cells (BFU-E) has also been recorded, the latter partly supported also by in vivo findings [3]; whether such activity is direct or is mediated by a cascade effect is still unclear. Besides acting on immature cells, G-CSF also modulates several functions of polymorphonuclear neutrophils (PMN), including enhancement of antibody-dependent cytotoxicity (ADCC), phagocytosis, superoxide generation and expression of f-Met-Leu-Phe-receptors [2, 4–11]. This factor has also been shown to be a chemotactic signal for phagocytes [12]. Finally, in contrast with GM-CSF, G-CSF does not induce the expression of surface glycoproteins associated with cell adhesion [2]. GM-CSF displays a broader effect on haematopoietic precursor cells than G-CSF, being active on pluripotent progenitors (CFU-GM), monocyte progenitors (CFU-M), eosinophil progenitors (CFU-Eo), megakaryociytic progenitors (CFU-Meg) and BFU-E [13]. In addition to regulating progenitor cell growth and differentiation, GM-CSF also has important effects on survival and function of mature myeloid cells. Its effects on neutrophil functions are essentially similar to those previously reported for G-CSF, including prolongation of survival, increased protein synthesis and chemotaxis, priming for degranulation, enhanced oxidative metabolism, increased release of arachidonic acid and leukotriene B4 and enhanced ADCC [13, 14]. Unlike G-CSF, GM-CSF has the capacity of inhibiting neutrophil migration due to the induction of surface antigen CD-11b; the frequent observation of a rapid fall in leukocyte counts after initiation of GM-CSF administration may indeed be interpreted as a consequence of leukocyte endothelium interactions caused by expression of the above-mentioned antigen [16]. As well as acting on neutrophils, GM-CSF also acts on eosinophils by prolonging in vitro survival, increasing ADCC and priming for leukotriene 4 release, and on mononuclear phagocytes by enhancing cytotoxicity, intracellular killing, phagocytosis and antigen processing [13].

With these biological properites, G-CSF and GM-CSF may be valuable therapeutic tools in clinical situations requiring accelerated proliferation of the haematopoietic lineages, rapid immunologic reconstitution, and enhanced defence against both infective agents and tumour cells, all aspects obviously of utmost importance in the setting of BMT.

Autologous Bone Marrow Transplantation

Most studies so far performed with G-CSF and GM-CSF in BMT have centered on autologous, rather than allogeneic transplantation, owing to the concern that these factors might exacerbate graft versus host disease (GVHD).

GM-CSF. Recombinant human GM-CSF (rHuGM-CSF) was the first HGF to be used in ABMT, after initial studies in patients with acquired immunodeficiency syndrome and myelodysplastic syndromes, that demonstrated a dose-dependent response of leukocyte counts [17, 18].

In a phase I/II study, rHuGM-CSF was given in escalating doses as a 2-hour daily infusion over 14 days to patients who had previously undergone ABMT for lymphoid malignancies [20]. The rHuGM-CSF effect turned out to be dose-related: most patients receiving >60 μg/m^2/day achieved an absolute neutrophil count $>0.5 \times 10/l$ before day 14, a significantly shorter period than recorded in the group of historical control patients, and became independent of platelet transfusions sooner. In patients treated with rHuGM-CSF >60 μg/m^2/day, the average number of days with temperature $>38\,°C$ as well as the number of days in hospital were also significantly reduced, indicating that acceleration of haematopoietic recovery after ABMT may result in a more favourable clinical course and saving of medical care costs, due to shorter hospital stay and less need for antibiotics. Finally, rHuGM-CSF treatment was well tolerated at doses up to 240 μg/m^2/day with only minor side effects such as muscle cramps and bone pain.

The efficacy of rHuGM-CSF in promoting haematopoietic recovery after ABMT has been proved also in patients with Hodgkin's disease [21]. In this series, however, no consistent effect on platelet counts was seen, and no difference could be detected between control and treated patients as far as rate of bacterial infections, number of febrile days and length of hospitalization were concerned.

Recently, interesting data have been published on the efficacy of rHuGM-CSF in ABMT for acute lymphoblastic leukaemia after previous in vitro purging with 4-hydroperoxycyclophosphamide and anti-T/anti-B antibodies, a procedure frequently leading to a reduction in the CFU-GM content of the transplanted marrow [22]. This study confirmed the efficacy of rHuGM-CSF in accelerating haematopoietic recovery, provided the factor is given at doses >60 µg/kg/day. In adequately treated patients, the response to rHuGM-CSF was significantly associated with the number of CFU-GM infused per kilogram, suggesting the need, when performing in vitro purging, for preserving a sufficient number of haematopoietic progenitors in the bone marrow.

rHuGM-CSF has been used in patients receiving high-dose chemotherapy and ABMT not only for haematological malignancies, but also for solid tumours. In a phase I trial, patients with refractory breast cancer and melanoma treated with combination chemotherapy and ABMT received rHuGM-CSF by continuous intravenous infusion for 14 days after BMT, at doses ranging from 2 to 32 µg/kg/day [23]. In these patients, total leukocyte and granulocyte recovery occurred more quickly than in historical controls matched for age, diagnosis and treatment. No consistent effect on platelet counts was recorded, and therefore, although GM-CSF has the ability to stimulate multilineage haematopoietic precursor cells in vitro, its principal target in this treatment setting seems to be the bipotential progenitor committed to granulocyte and macrophage production. After discontinuation of rHuGM-CSF administration, leukocyte counts fell for a period of 3–4 days to the level ordinarily expected after transplantation, and then rose at a rate comparable to that in historical controls. This finding of a prompt fall in cell counts, as well as the rapid increase of cells at the start of treatment, may indeed indicate that rHuGm-CSF might have additional effects also on marrow release, margination and extravascular distribution of leukocytes. A further interesting finding of this study was that rHuGM-CSF-treated patients had less hepatotoxicity and nephrotoxicity than controls, possibly related to a lower frequency of bacterial complications. Whereas toxicity at doses of 2–16 µg/kg/day was mild, not clearly dose-related and reversible upon discontinuation of rHuGM-CSF, at the dose of 32 µg/kg/day side effects were severe, consisting of erythroderma, weight gain, generalized edema, pleural effusion and hypotension, probably caused by a capillary leak syndrome similar to the one associated with high-dose interleukin-2 therapy [24].

Further pilot studies in patients undergoing ABMT for solid tumours have confirmed the beneficial effects of rHuGM-CSF on leukocyte recovery [25].

G-CSF. The use of G-CSF in ABMT has now been reported in several studies and the overall results strongly support a significant reduction of the period of chemotherapy-related neutropenia. In a series of patients undergoing ABMT for high-risk acute lymphoblastic leukaemia, non-Hodgkin's lymphomas and germ-cell tumours, rHuG-CSF at a starting dose of 20 µg/kg/day was given as a continuous infusion until neutrophil counts reached 1.5×10/l [26]. The mean time to neutrophil recovery was significantly less than in the matched historical control group. The need for parenteral antibiotics, as well as the length of hospitalization, days of parenteral nutrition and days of isolation were also significantly reduced in rHuG-CSF-treated patients. Adverse reactions possibly related to therapy were limited to the infrequent appearance of erythema at subcutaneous infusion sites. Similar results were reported in patients with relapsed or refractory Hodgkin's disease treated with cytotoxic therapy followed by ABMT who received rHuG-CSF either by continuous infusion or bolus injection at doses between 30 and 120 µg/kg/day for up to 28 days post ABMT. In both instances, the period required for neutrophil recovery was significantly shorter than in the control group; the treated group experienced also fewer febrile days and a lower rate of gram-positive infections. Toxicity was mild and transient, consisting of myalgias and bone pain. The efficacy of rHuG-CSF after ABMT has been proved also in advanced breast cancer and advanced melanoma [28].

Allogeneic Bone Marrow Transplantation

As previously stated, the use of HGFs in allogeneic BMT has so far been limited owing to concern that they might stimulate cells responsible for graft failure or graft-versus-host disease.

Preliminary results, however, suggest that HGFs in allogeneic BMT can improve marrow recovery without increasing the risk of graft-versus-host disease [29, 30].

In a phase II study, rHuG-CSF was given as bolus injection at doses ranging from 200 to 800 μg/m^2 after allogeneic BMT in patients with haematological malignancies [30]. A faster granulocyte recovery was observed in treated patients, which was not associated with consistent effects on lymphocyte, eosinophil and platelet counts; the incidence of relapse, frequency and severity of GVHD were apparently not affected by rHuG-CSF administration.

Peripheral Stem Cell Transplantation

The finding that injection of either G-CSF or GM-CSF can markedly increase the number of circulating peripheral blood haematopoietic progenitors has generated interest in the use of HGFs for facilitating the harvesting of peripheral blood stem cells for autotransplantation [31, 32]. To this aim, GM-CSF was used in association with cyclophosphamide in patients with non-Hodgkin's lymphomas [33]. During the recovery phase, patients underwent leucapheresis with an about nine-fold increased yield of CFU-GM compared with a control group. Previously harvested autologous bone marrow and peripheral stem cells were then successfully reinfused after a conditioning regimen with melphalan and total body irradiation.

Graft Failure

Although sustained engraftment is the rule after BMT, in some cases, patients either fail to engraft or the graft ceases to function after a period of normal activity. Two different types of graft failure are presently recognized. Graft rejection, which is seen in about 2% of allogeneic BMT, is thought to be caused by immunocompetent host cells surviving the conditioning regimen and reacting with unshared antigenic determinants expressed on donor cells.

True graft failure seems to be due not to immunocompetent effector cells but to damage of the marow prior to transplantation, to viral infections such as cytomegalovirus or to untoward drug reactions.

Since treatments for graft rejection or failure are usually poorly effective, attention has been given to the possible therapeutic role of HGFs in this clinical setting. In a phase I–II trial, patients with graft failure were treated with rHuGM-CSF by 2-hour infusion of escalating doses starting at 60 μg/m^2/day for 14 days and increasing to 1,000 μg/m^2 [34]. An increase of granulocyte counts above 500/mm^3 was recorded in about half of the patients without a concomitant effect on platelet and erythrocyte counts. The granulocyte response persisted also after stopping treatment. RHuGM-CSF was well tolerated at doses up to 250 μg/m^2, whereas at 500 μg/m^2 and over, it caused fever, bone pain and abdominal cramps, and in 1 case also pericarditis.

Problems Related to the Use of G-CSF and GM-CSF in BMT

Effects on Leukaemic Cells

Whereas both GM-CSF and G-CSF have been found to stimulate in vitro proliferation and self-renewal of blast cells from acute non-lymphocytic leukaemias [35, 36], the clinical use of these factors in myelodysplastic syndromes (MDS) has yielded conflicting results as far as stimulation of blast cells is concerned. In one study on MDS including also refractory anaemia with excess of blasts in transformation, no increase in absolute blast counts was recorded, whereas in other trials on the same type of patients, GM-CSF induced an increase of marrow myeloblasts [37–39]. On the other hand G-CSF, so far scarcely used in myelodysplastic syndromes, seems to have no stimulatory effect on leukaemia cells. Although GM-CSF stimulation of blast cells can obviously be viewed as an untoward side effect causing expansion of a malignant population, it might also be taken as a potential benefit in that leukaemia cells are recruited into the cell cycle and thus rendered more sensitive to cycle-specific cytotoxic agents. Preliminary data support the efficacy of this combined therapeutic approach [41].

Effects on Non-Haematopoietic Malignant Cells

Due to the increasing use of CSFs to reconstitute bone marrow of tumour patients following chemotherapy and BMT, the growth-modulating effects of CSFs on cancer cells has become a crucial aspect. GM-CSF receptors have been reported in several solid tumours such as sarcomas, breast cancer and small-cell lung cancer [42, 43]. The importance of this finding is however uncertain since, for instance, GM-CSF has been variously reported to stimulate, inhibit and have no effect on the growth of cell lines derived from small-cell lung cancer [44–46]. In a series of cancer patients treated also with GM-CSF, however, the response rate and durability of responses were similar to those in historical controls, apparently ruling out an untoward GM-CSF effect on neoplastic growth [23].

On the other hand, as reported above for leukaemia, stimulation of tumour cell proliferation by CSFs may also be viewed as a tool for enhancing sensitivity to cytotoxic chemotherapy, but clinical trials on this therapeutic approach have not yet been performed in solid tumours.

Effects on Phagocyte and Neutrophil Function

As mentioned above, in vivo GM-CSF administration has been shown to cause transient leucopenia due to increased expression of cell surface adherence molecules followed by margination caused by endothelial adherence [15]. Such margination may have important clinical consequences at specific anatomic sites, since, for instance, signs of pulmonary consolidation have been reported in patients with preexisting lung diseases treated with GM-CSF [47, 48].

GM-CSF has also been shown to inhibit neutrophil migration significantly, thus impairing an adequate response to an appropriate signal from an inflammatory focus [49, 50]; caution should therefore be used in protracting GM-CSF administration in patients with severe, deep-seated infections.

Conclusion

Although still at an early stage, clinical investigations on the role of G-CSF and GM-CSF in BMT seem to indicate a clear-cut effect in accelerating leucocyte and neutrophil recovery. Disappointingly, the efficacy of GM-CSF on platelet regeneration, which might have been predicted based on its in vitro activity, is at the moment inconsistent.

According to some trials, accelerated haematopoietic recovery after BMT results in a clinical benefit owing to less infections, reduced use of antibiotics and blood components, and decreased length of hospital stay. However, larger randomized clinical studies still seem required to address the issue of the impact of CSFs treatment on morbidity, mortality and quality of life of patients undergoing BMT.

Finally, it can be envisaged that an optimal use of haematopoietic growth factors, by allowing fast marrow reconstitution after anticancer therapy, might ultimately lead to a less frequent need for BMT, which has to be viewed as a supportive procedure presently required to overcome major haematological toxicity caused by high-dose anti-tumour treatment.

References

1 Souza LM, Boone TC, Gabrilove J, Lai PH, Zsebo KM, Murdock DC, Chazin VR, Bruszewski J, Lu H, Chen KK, Barendt E, Moore MAS, Mertelsmann R, Welte K: Recombinant human granulocyte colony-stimulating factor: Effects on normal and leukemic myeloid cells. Science 1986;232:61–65.
2 Lindemann A, Herrmann F, Oster W, Haffner G, Meyenburg W, Souza LM, Mertelsmann R: Haematologic effects of recombinant human granulocyte colony stimulating factor in patients with malignancy. Blood 1989;74:2644–2657.
3 Sieff CA: Haematopoietic growth factors. J Clin Invest 1987; 79:1549–1557.
4 Platzer E, Welte K, Gabrilove JC, Harris T, Mertelsmann R, Moore MAS: Biological activities of a pluripotent haematopoietic colony stimulating factor on normal and leukemic cells. J Exp Med 1985;162:1788–1801.
5 Platzer E, Oez S, Welte K, Sendler A, Gabrilove JL, Mertelsmann R, Moore MAS, Kalden JR: Human pluripotent hematopoietic colony stimulating factor: Activities on human and murine cells. Immunobiology 1986;172:185–193.
6 Weisbart RH, Gasson JC, Golde DW: Colony-stimulating factors and host defense. Ann Intern Med 1989;110:279–303.
7 Weisbart RH, Golde DW, Clark SC, Wong GG, Gasson JC: Human granulocyte-macrophage colony stimulating factor is a neutrophil activator. Nature 1985;314:361–363.
8 Weisbart RH, Golde DW, Gasson JC: Biosynthetic human GM-CSF modulates the number and affinity of neutrophil-Met-Leu-Phe-receptors. J Immunol 1986;137:3584–3587.
9 Weisbart RH, Kacena A, Shuh A, Golde DW: GM-CSF induces human neutrophil IgA-mediated phagogytosis by an IgA Fc-receptor activation mechanism. Nature 1988;332:467–648.
10 Weisbart RH, Kwan L, Golde DW, Gasson JC: Human GM-CSF primes neutrophils for enhanced oxidative metabolism in response to the major physiological chemoattractants. Blood 1987;69:18–21.
11 Welte K, Bonilla MA, Gillio AP, Boone TC, Potter GK, Gabrilove JL, Moore MAS, O'Reilly RD, Souza LM: Recombinant human granulocyte colony stimulating factor: Effects on hematopoiesis in normal and cyclophosphamide treated primates. J Exp Med 1987;165:941–948.
12 Wang JM, Chen ZG, Golella S, Bonilla MA, Welte K, Bordignon C, Mantovani A: Chemotactic activity of recombinant G-CSF. Blood 1988;72:1456–1460.
13 Golde DW: Overview of myeloid growth factors. Semin Haematol 1990;27:1–7.
14 Golde DW, Baldwin GC, Weisbart RH: Response of neutrophils to myeloid growth factors; in Molecular Control of Haematopoiesis. Proc CIBA Symp No 148. New York, Wiley, 1990, pp 62–75.
15 Arnaout MA, Wang EA, Clark SC, Sieff CA: Human recombinant granulocyte-macrophage colony-stimulating factor increases cell-to-cell adhesion and surface expression of adhe-

sion-promoting surface glycoproteins on mature granulocytes. J Clin Invest 1986;78:597–601.
16 Herrmann F, Schulz G, Lindemann A, Meyenburg W, Oster W, Krumwieh D, Mertelsmann R: Hematopoietic responses in patients with advanced malignancy treated with recombinant human granulocyte macrophage colony-stimulating factor. J Clin Oncol 1989;7:159–167.
17 Groopman JE, Mitsuyasu RT, DeLeo MJ, Oette DH, Golde DW: Effect of recombinant human granulocyte-macrophage colony-stimulating factor on myelopoiesis in the acquired immunodeficiency syndrome. N Engl J Med 1987;317:593–598.
18 Vadhan-Raj S, Keating M, Le Maistre A, Hittelmann WN, McCredie K, Trujillo JM, Broxmeyer HE, Henney C, Guttermann JU: Effects of recombinant human granulocyte macrophage colony stimulating factor in patients with myelodysplastic syndromes. N Engl J Med 1987;317:1545–1552.
19 Peters WP: The effects of recombinant human colony-stimulating factors on haematopoietic reconstitution following autologous bone marrow transplantation. Semin Haematol 1988; 26(suppl 2):18–23.
20 Nemunaitis J, Singer JW, Buckner CD, et al: Use of recombinant human granulocyte-macrophage colony-stimulating factor in autologous marrow transplantation for lymphoid malignancies. Blood 1988;72:834–836.
21 Devereux S, Linch DC, Gribben JG, McMillan A, Patterson K, Goldstone AH: GM-CSF accelerates neutrophil recovery after autologous bone marrow transplantation for Hodgkin's disease. Bone Marrow Transplant 1989;4:49–54.
22 Blazar BR, Kersey JH, McGlave PB, et al: In vivo administration of recombinant human granulocyte-macrophage colony-stimulating factor in acute lymphoblastic leukemia patients receiving purged autografts. Blood 1989;73:849–857.
23 Fouillard L, Isnard F, Najaman A: Recombinant granulocyte-macrophage colony-stimulating factor after BEAM regimen instead of autologous bone marrow transplantation (letter). Lancet 1989;i:1360.
24 Rosestein R, Ettinghausen SE, Rosenberg SA: Extravasation of intravascular fluid mediated by systemic administration of recombinant interleukin-2. J Immunol 1986;137:1735–1742.
25 Link H, Burdach S, Seidel J, et al: Recombinant human granulocyte-macrophage colony-stimulating factor after autologous bone marrow transplantation (abstract No 23). Mol Biother 1989;1(suppl):8.
26 Sheridan WP, Wolf M, Lusk J, et al: Granulocyte colony-stimulating factor and neutrophil recovery after high-dose chemotherapy and autologous bone marrow transplantation. Lancet 1989;ii:891–895.
27 Taylor K, Jagannath S, Spizer G, et al: Recombinant human granulocyte colony-stimulating factor hastens granulocyte recovery after high-dose chemotherapy and autologous bone marrow transplantation in Hodgkin's disease. J Clin Oncol, in press.
28 Peters W: The effect of recombinant human colony-stimulating factors on hematopoietic reconstitution following autologous bone marrow transplantation. Semin Haematol 1989; 26(suppl 2):18–23.
29 Nemunaitis J, Singer JW, Buckner CD, et al: The use of rHuGM-CSF for graft failure in patients after autologous allogeneic, or syngeneic bone marrow transplantation (BMT) (abstract No 1503). Blood 1988;72(suppl 1):398A.
30 Nasaoka T: Recombinant human granulocyte colony-stimulating factor in allogeneic bone marrow transplantation. Exp Haematol 1989;17:1047–1050.
31 Duhrsen U, Villeval JL, Boyd J, Kannourakis G, Morstyn G, Metcalf D: Effcts of recombinant human granulocyte colony-stimulating factor on hematopoietic progenitor cells in cancer patients. Blood 1988;72:2074–2081.
32 Socinski MA, Cannistra SA, Elias A, Antman KH, Schnipper L, Griffin JD: Granulocyte-macrophage colony-stimulating factor expands the circulating hematopoietic progenitor cell compartment in man. Lancet 1988;i:1194.
33 Gianni AM, Siena S, Bregni M, Tarella C, Stern AC, Pileri A, Bonadonna G: Granulocyte-macrophage colony-stimulating factor to harvest circulating haematopoietic stem cells for autotransplantation. Lancet 1989;ii:580.
34 Nemunaitis J, Singer JW, Buckner CD, et al: The use of RhGM-CSF for graft failure in patients after autologous, allogeneic bone marrow transplantation (BMT). Blood 1988;72: 398a.
35 Hoang T, Nara N, Wong G, Clark S, Minden MD, McColloch EA: Effects of recombinant GM-CSF on the blast cells of acute myeloblastic leukaemia. Blood 1986;68:313–316.
36 Miyauchi J, Kelleher CA, Yang YC, Wong GG, Clark SC, Minden MD, Minkin S, McCulloch EA: The effects of three recombinant growth factors, IL-3, GM-CSF, and G-CSF, on the blast cells of acute myeloblastic leukaemia maintained in short-term suspension culture. Blood 1987;70:657–663.
37 Antin JH, Smith BR, Holmes W, Rosenthal DS: Phase I/II study of recombinant human granulocyte-macrophage colony-stimulating factor in aplastic anemia and myelodysplastic syndrome. Blood 1988;72:705–713.
38 Ganser A, Volkers B, Greher J, Ottman OG, Walther F, Becher R, Bergmann L, Schulz G, Hoelzer D: Recombinant human granulocyte-macrophage colony-stimulating factor in patients with myelodysplastic syndromes – a phase I/II trial. Blood 1989;73:31–37.
39 Negrin RS, Haeuber DH, Nagler A, Olds LC, Donlon T, Souza LM, Greenberg PL: Treatment of myelodysplastic syndromes with recombinant human granulocyte colony-stimulating factor. Ann Intern Med 1989;110:976–984.
40 Ganser A, Hoelzer D: Recombinant human granulocyte-macrophage colony stimulating factor and low-dose cytosine arabinoside in patients with myelodysplastic syndromes. Onkologie 1989;12:13–15.
41 Baldwin GC: Characterization of human GM-CSF receptors on non-hematopoietic cells. Blood 1987;68:166a.
42 De Dhar S: Human granulocyte-macrophage colony stimulating factor is a growth factor for a variety of cell types of non-hematopoietic origin. 79th Annual ASCO Meet, New Orleans, 1988, p 51a.
43 Baldwin GC, DiuPersio J, Kaufmann SE, Quan SG, Golde DW, Gassor JC: Characterization of human GM-CSF receptors on non-hematopoietic cells (abstract). Blood 1987;70:166a.
44 Ruff MR, Farrar WL, Pert CB: Interferon γ and granulocyte macrophage colony stimulating factor inhibit growth and induce antigens characteristic of myeloid differentiation in small-cell lung cancer cell lines. Proc Natl Acad Sci USA 1986; 83:6613–6617.
45 Munker M, Munker R, Saxton RE, Koeffler HP: Effect of recombinant monokines, lymphokines and other agents on clo-

nal proliferation of human lung cancer cell lines. Cancer Res 1987;47:4081–4085.

46 Devereux S, Linch DC, Gribben JG, McMillan A, Patterson K, Goldstone AH: GM-CSF accelerates neutrophil recovery after autologous bone marrow transplantation for Hodgkin's disease. Bone Marrow Transplant 1989;4:49–54.

47 Champlin RE, Nimer SD, Ireland P, Oette DH, Golde DW: Treatment of refractory aplastic anemia with recombinant human granulocyte-macrophage colony-stimulating factor. Blood 1989;73:694–699.

48 Addison IE, Johnson B, Devereux S, Goldstone AH, Linch DC: Granulocyte macrophage colony-stimulating factor may inhibit neutrophil migration in vivo. Clin Exp Immunol 1989; 76:149–153.

49 Peters WP, Stuart A, Affronti ML, Kim CS, Coleman RE: Neutrophil migration is defective during recombinant granulocyte-macrophage colony-stimulating factor infusion after autologous bone marrow transplantation in humans. Blood 1988; 72:1310–1315.

E.E. Polli, MD
Istituto di Scienze Mediche
Padiglione Granelli
Via F. Sforza 35
I–20122 Milano (Italy)

Acta Haematol 1991;86:162–168

Erythropoietin: Clinical Applications

P. Foa

Istituto di Scienze Mediche, Padiglione Granelli, Milano, Italia

Key Words. Anaemia associated with cancer · Anaemia associated with myelodysplastic syndromes · Anaemia of AIDS · Anaemia of renal disease · Autotransfusion · Erythropoietin · Haematopoietic growth factors

Abstract. The last few years have seen an enormous increase in our knowledge on the haematopoietic growth factor erythropoietin (Epo), firstly with its purification and determination of its primary amino acid sequence, and more recently with the isolation of the Epo gene and its expression in mammalian cell lines. This review article summarizes the crucial biological features of Epo and critically examines the main results obtained in clinical trials on humans.

Introduction

Although it is presently recognized that proliferation and differentiation of the erythroid lineage can be affected by several endogenous molecules [1], erythropoietin (Epo) still stands as the primary physiological regulator of erythropoiesis. Mostly due to the identification of the Epo amino acid sequence, the isolation of the Epo gene and, finally, its expression in mammalian cell lines, in the last few years the knowledge of this factor has increased enormously [2–5].

Epo is an acidic, heat-stable, single-chain glycoprotein with a total molecular weight of 34,000 D [6, 7]; glycosylation is not essential for Epo biological activity, but helps to prevent fast hepatic clearance of the desialated form [8].

The Epo gene, which shows no homology with any other known gene, is a single-copy gene located on the long arm of chromosome 7 in region 21 [3, 4, 9]. Epo production is controlled by the modulation of a 1.8-kb mRNA, which increases following a hypoxic stimulus due to enhanced gene expression [10, 11].

The main Epo production site in post-fetal life is in the kidney, namely, peritubular cells outside the tubular basement membrane where a specific 1.8-kb mRNA has recently been identified [12, 13]. A close correlation seems to exist between haematocrit and number of Epo-producing cells, thus suggesting that an increase of Epo synthesis is achieved by recruiting basally quiescent cells for production, in addition to increasing the synthetic activity of single cells. Quite recently, it has been shown that the Epo gene is expressed also in bone marrow macrophages [14]; this finding agrees well with the widely accepted concept that regulation of haematopoiesis also depends upon humoral interactions within the bone marrow microenvironment.

Epo exerts its physiological activity by controlling the proliferation, differentiation and maturation of erythroid progenitors [1, 15–18]. Two different types of erythroid progenitors, one more immature (burst-forming unit erythroid, BFU-E) and the other more mature (colony-forming unit erythroid, CFU-E), are presently recognized [19, 20]; transition from BFU-E to CFU-E is characterized by higher proliferative activity and increasing sensitivity to Epo so that, whereas the activity of BFU-E is affected by a number of non-Epo haematopoietic growth factors such as IL-3, G-CSF and GM-CSF, at the CFU-E stage cells are largely dependent on Epo for growth and development into erythroid mature cells [21–25].

Based on recent findings, it has been suggested that Epo can also affect target cells other than those of the erythroid lineage, such as megakaryocyte precursors (CFU-Meg), granulocyte-macrophage colony-forming units (CFU-GM) and the pluripotent stem cell (CFU-GEMM) [26–28]; however, it is as yet unclear whether such a multilineage effect is direct or mediated by secondary factors.

Like other protein hormones, Epo exerts its biological activity through a receptor-mediated mechanism. Both high- and low-affinity receptors have been identified [29–31], which are presumed to differ as far as function is concerned. Namely, high-affinity receptors seem to be required for Epo-induced erythroid differentiation, whereas low-affinity ones seem to be involved in the proliferative effects of Epo [32, 33].

Clinical Use

As previously mentioned, the successful cloning and expression of the human Epo gene has made recombinant human Epo (rHuEpo) available not only for biological investigation but also for exploring the therapeutic usefulness of this factor.

In the next paragraphs, the main results obtained with the clinical use of rHuEpo will be reviewed.

Anaemia of Renal Disease

The therapeutic efficacy of rHuEpo was first evaluated in patients with end-stage renal disease, a clinical setting frequently complicated by severe anaemia which often impairs rehabilitation despite adequate dialysis therapy and requires red cell transfusions. The mechanism underlying this type of anaemia is complex, probably involving shortening of red cell survival, inhibition of erythropoiesis, iron deficiency, hypersplenism and aluminium-induced microcytosis, but a primary role is certainly played by impaired Epo production in the damaged kidneys [34–38].

In late 1986 and 1987, the results of the initial phase I and II clinical trials with rHuEpo in severely anaemic patients on chronic haemodialysis (HD) were reported [39, 40]. The hormone was given intravenously, three times weekly following each HD, at doses from 1.5 to 500 IU/kg. A dose- and time-related increase of reticulocytes and haematocrit was recorded, and correction of anaemia and disappearance of blood transfusions requirement was achieved in the majority of patients receiving effective dosages. Elimination of transfusion requirement obviously represents a major improvement for these patients, who thus avoid the risk of iron overload, exposure to infective agents and alloimmunization.

These encouraging results have been confirmed by a number of studies all showing the efficacy of rHuEpo treatment in this type of anaemia [41–48]. As expected, normalization of haemoglobin levels results also in improvement of the well-being of HD patients and of their cardiac and respiratory function, exercise capacity, and sexual activity [49–52]. Moreover, the effectiveness of rHuEpo treatment has been demonstrated by ferrokinetic studies, which showed a 2- to 4-fold increase of erythropoietic activity with respect to pretreatment values [53, 54]. Such an rHuEpo-driven increase of haemoglobin synthesis, often exceeding the capacity of the reticuloendothelial system to release iron to transferrin, may result in a state of functional iron deficiency requiring adequate oral or intravenous iron supplementation [39].

In some rHuEpo-treated patients, ‘in vitro’ assessments of haematopoietic progenitor cell activity have also been performed. In addition to the expected increase of CFU-E, an increase of BFU-E as well as of CFU-Meg and CFU-GM was also recorded, which however did not result in a significant change of leukocyte counts in peripheral blood [55, 56]. Data on platelet counts in rHuEpo-treated patients are more conflicting since they have sometimes been found to be unaffected and sometimes significantly increased [57]; whether this latter effect actually reflects an influence of rHuEpo on CFU-Meg or is attributable to reactive thrombocytosis induced by relative iron deficiency is still unclear.

In the above-mentioned studies of patients with end-stage renal disease, no important toxic effects, allergic reactions or antibody formation were observed. However, the adaptation of previously anaemic patients to an increase in red-cell mass and blood viscosity has sometimes generated a rise of blood pressure, rarely associated with seizures, requiring the institution or increase of antihypertensive treatment.

In addition to rHuEpo-induced changes of the red-cell mass, this phenomenon seems to be attributable also to loss of the vasodilatatory effect caused by anaemia-dependent hypoxia, rather than to a direct vasoconstrictive activity of rHuEpo [58, 59]. Careful monitoring of blood pressure in rHuEpo treated patients is therefore warranted, especially during the initial phase of treatment. Finally, conflicting results have been reported on the incidence of clotting of vascular access for HD in rHuEpo-treated patients [57, 60, 61].

Recently, the therapeutic efficacy of rHuEpo has

been assessed also in patients with chronic renal insufficiency not yet requiring HD; essentially the same type of findings as previously reported for HD patients have been obtained [62, 64].

An issue which has still to be fully clarified as far as the therapeutic use of rHuEpo is concerned, is the optimal dosage and mode of administration. According to recent findings, the high peaks obtained after intravenous administration of rHuEpo are unnecessary for its efficacy, suggesting that the subcutaneous route, with which more persistent although lower rHuEpo blood levels are obtained, might be the elective route of administration for this factor [65–68].

Autotransfusion in Surgical Settings

A further area of interest for the clinical use of rHuEpo is autologous blood donation, the safest transfusional procedure for elective surgery. It is well known that candidates for elective surgery are often unable to donate the necessary amount of blood owing to the development of phlebotomy-related anaemia, and therefore require also homologous blood supply. Recent studies have shown that such an anaemia is likely due to an inadequate increase of the endogenous Epo response, insufficient to stimulate compensatory bone marrow erythropoiesis [69–70]. These findings suggest that administration of rHuEpo might prevent the development of anaemia in such patients and increase the volume of autologous blood that can be collected before surgery. It is also conceivable that pretreatment of surgical patients with rHuEpo, by stimulating bone marrow proliferation, might result in more effective compensation for surgical blood loss and reduce the need for red cell transfusion during both the operative and postoperative periods.

The results of preliminary studies designed to clarify the actual role of rHuEpo treatment in this clinical setting have recently been published [71, 72]. About 40% more red cells could be collected from patients receiving rHuEpo than from the placebo-treated group, and the requirement for homologous blood was consequently less; no adverse effects related to rHuEpo administration were observed. Although larger series are required to confirm these preliminary data, it seems predictable that adjunctive therapy with rHuEpo will become increasingly important for programs of autologous blood donation in surgical settings.

Anaemia of Rheumatoid Arthritis

The pathogenesis of anaemia in rheumatoid arthritis (RA) is multifactorial, including altered ferrokinetics and slightly reduced red cell life span as well as impaired bone marrow response to high levels of endogenous Epo [73]. This defective response to Epo seems to be attributable not only to the reduced release of iron from the reticuloendothelial system but mostly to high levels of interleukin 1, a cytokine that is produced in increased amounts by blood mononuclear cells in RA patients and has recently been shown to inhibit the growth of erythroid cells in vitro [74–77]. Preliminary clinical trials have therefore been performed in order to assess whether administration of adequate amounts of rHuEpo might be able to correct the defective marrow response reported in this type of anaemia. Adequately treated patients have presented increases of haematocrit values, red cell mass and bone marrow erythroid progenitor cells [78, 79]; it is however as yet unclear whether the quality of life and/or joint symptoms will also improve as a result of rHuEpo administration.

While more data are necessary before firm conclusions can be drawn on the therapeutic utility of rHuEpo in RA, it is encouraging that also anaemia of chronic inflammatory disease appears responsive to rHuEpo.

Anaemia Associated with Malignancy

Anaemia is a frequent finding in cancer patients, even before they receive cytotoxic chemotherapy. While factors such as bone marrow infiltration by neoplastic cells, haemorrhage, poor nutrition and autoimmune and microangiopathic haemolysis, certainly contribute to this type of anaemia, the haematological picture in this setting is often similar to the anaemia of chronic disorders, namely an underproduction anaemia in the presence of increased Epo levels [80].

Like RA patients who often have high levels of the cytokine interleukin 1, so also cancer patients frequently present increased serum levels of a powerful inhibitor of erythropoiesis, tumor necrosis factor (TNF) [81–83]. Moreover, it has recently been demonstrated that in cancer patients with any given degree of anaemia, the serum concentrations of Epo, while increased, are however lower than in a group of control patients with iron deficiency anaemia, thus suggesting that Epo production is inadequate in cancer patients [84]. Based on these observations, rHuEpo has been given to anaemic cancer patients with the aim of correcting defective erythropoiesis. Most of the clinical data so far available have been obtained in patients with lymphoproliferative diseases, namely low-grade non-Hodgkin's lymphomas and multiple myeloma with anaemia due to neoplastic bone marrow infiltration [85, 86]. Despite high basal levels of endogenous Epo, exogenous administration of rHuEpo in pharmacological concentrations caused a significant rise of haemoglobin, haematocrit and erythrocyte counts in most patients. Initial serum ferritin values, which were usually high owing to multiple transfusions, were significantly reduced as a consequence of iron overconsumption by stimulated erythropoiesis. Interestingly, increased platelet counts were also recorded in a few patients [85]; no important adverse events due to rHuEpo administration were observed.

Although anaemia in patients with cancer is seldom the main factor in their symptoms and morbidity, response to treatment with rHuEpo resulted in an improved quality of life and performance status.

A further possible role for rHuEpo treatment in cancer patients is related to the frequent occurrence of anaemia due to chemotherapy regimens. According to preliminary data, rHuEpo administered to patients undergoing chemotherapy can maintain haemoglobin at above 9 g/dl, thus obviating the need for erythrocyte transfusion [87]. In addition to the rise of haemoglobin, a significant reduction of serum ferritin was observed, a further sign of stimulated erythropoiesis.

As a whole, clinical data so far available suggest that rHuEpo, by supporting and stimulating erythropoiesis, may have a valuable role in the treatment of selected cancer patients.

Anaemia Associated with Myelodysplastic Syndromes

Myelodysplastic syndromes (MDS) are a heterogeneous group of haematological disorders characterized by ineffective haematopoiesis, refractory cytopenia and frequent progression to overt acute leukaemia. So far, treatment approaches based on the use of conventional cytostatic agents or differentiation-inducing compounds have met with little success, and usually no overall survival advantage has been achieved in comparison with supportive therapy alone.

Since normal bone marrow cells can coexist together with abnormal cells in early stages of MDS, it has been speculated that Epo might provide a growth advantage for normal residual haematopoiesis, thus reducing the degree of anaemia and the transfusion requirement. In addition, since the abnormal clone of MDS might still retain its sensitivity to haematopoietic growth factors, it has also been suggested that pharmacological levels of Epo might force cellular differentiation towards mature terminal cells.

Despite consistent in vitro experimental data indicating that MDS-derived haematopoietic bone marrow cells respond poorly to some cytokines and fail to show adequate growth [88, 89], clinical trials have been performed to assess the possible therapeutic role of rHuEpo in MDS.

Data so far available are both scanty and conflicting. While in a few patients an increase of absolute reticulocyte number and haemoglobin levels has been achieved with a concomitant reduction of the blood transfusion requirement [90, 92], most often rHuEpo administration in MDS patients has led only to minor changes of peripheral blood values with little impact on the actual need for supportive treatment.

This poor activity of rHuEpo might be related to the high basal level of endogenous Epo usually observed in MDS patients, suggesting that the anaemia of such disorders is actually due to dyserythropoiesis rather than to insufficient production of Epo itself [93]. However, more extensive data are required prior to making any definitive conclusions on the therapeutic role of rHuEpo in MDS.

Anaemia of AIDS Treated with Zidovudine

Zidovudine (AZT) has been reported to be an effective agent in reducing signs and symptoms of infection and in prolonging survival in AIDS patients. However, it can cause bone marrow suppression resulting in severe, transfusion-dependent anaemia. Assuming that AZT remains the most effective means for treating AIDS, and taking into account the estimated prevalence of this type of anaemia, the burden on blood transfusion services is going to be increased substantially. Moreover, blood transfusion has been shown to exert an immunosuppressive effect in a variety of clinical settings, and this might eventually affect the course of AIDS patients.

Based on these observations, prospective randomised clinical trials have been performed to evaluate the efficacy of rHuEpo administration in AIDS patients treated with AZT. Interestingly, it has been shown that AZT can induce two distinct types of anaemia, the first with macrocytosis, Epo endogenous serum levels lower than 500 IU/litre and moderate transfusion requirement, the second associated with normocytic red cells, Epo endogenous serum levels above 500 IU/litre and high transfusion requirement. According to the clinical data so far available, rHuEpo at the dose of 100 IU/kg body weight given thrice weekly by intravenous bolus is effective in significantly decreasing the blood transfusion requirement in patients with anaemia of the first type, but not in those with anaemia of the second type [93]. It is however possible that either with higher doses of rHuEpo or lower doses of AZT, also patients with high base-line endogenous Epo levels might also respond.

Conclusion

A survey of the clinical trials performed so far, clearly indicates that rHuEpo already has an established role in the treatment of anaemia associated with several diseases, as for instance end-stage renal insufficiency, RA and cancer with malignant bone marrow infiltration. Furthermore, rHuEpo has turned out to be useful also in specific clinical settings, such as autologous blood transfusion before elective surgery and prevention and/or treatment of anaemia induced by cytostatic drugs. Further experience is however required in order to clarify whether rHuEpo can be effective in diseases such as MDS and AIDS.

References

1 Graber SE, Krantz SB: Erythropoietin: Biology and clinical use. Hematol Oncol Clin North Am 1989;3:369–400.
2 Miyake T, Kung CKH, Goldwasser E: Purification of human erythropoietin. J Biol Chem 1977;252:5558–5564.
3 Jacobs K, Shoemaker C, Rudersdorf R: Isolation and characterization of genomic and cDNA clones of human erythropoietin. Nature 1985;313:806–809.
4 Lin FK, Suggs, Lin CH: Cloning and expression of the human erythropoietin gene. Proc Natl Acad Sci USA 1985;82:7580–7584.
5 Egrie JC, Strickland TW, Lane J: Characterization and biological effects of recombinant human erythropoietin. Immunobiology 1986;172:213–224.
6 Lai PH, Everett R, Wang FF, Arakawa T, Goldwasser E: Structural characterization of human erythropoietin. J Biol Chem 1986;261:3116–3121.
7 Hirth P, Weczorek L, Scigalla P: Molecular biology of erythropoietin; in Koch KM, Kuhn K, Nonnast-Daniel B, Scigalla P (eds): Treatment of renal anemia with recombinant human erythropoietin. Basel, Karger, 1988, pp 38–53.
8 Spivak JL, Hogans BB: The in vivo metabolism of recombinant human erythropoietin. Blood 1988;73:90–99.
9 Law ML, Cai GY, Lin FK: Chromosomal assignment of the human erythropoietin gene and its DNA polymorphism. Proc Natl Acad Sci USA 1986;83:6920–6924.
10 Shuster SJ, Wilson JH, Erslev AJ, Caro J: Physiologic regulation and tissue localization of renal erythropoietin messenger RNA. Blood 1987;70:316–318.
11 Shuster SJ, Badiavas EV, Costa-Giomi P, Weinmann Rm, Erslev AJ, Caro J: Stimulation of erythropoietin gene transcriptions during hypoxia and cobalt exposure. Blood 1989;73:13–16.
12 Koury ST, Bondurant MC, Koury MJ: Localization of erythropoietin synthesizing cells in murine kidney by in situ hybridizant. Blood 1988;71:524–527.
13 Lacombe C, Da Silva JL, Bruneval P: Peritubular cells are the site of erythropoietin synthesis in the murine hypoxic kidney. J Clin Invest 1988;81:620–623.
14 Vogt C, Pentz S, Rich I: A role for the macrophage in the normal hemopoiesis. III. In vitro and in vivo erythropoietin gene expression in macrophages detected by in situ hybridization. Exp Hematol 1989;17:391–397.
15 Spivak JL: Themechanism of action of erythropoietin. Int J Cell Cloning 1986;4:139–166.
16 Papayannopoulou T, Finch C: On the in vivo action of erythropoietin: A quantitative analysis. J Clin Invest 1972;51:1179–1185.
17 Hambley H, Mufty G: Erythropoietin: An old friend revisited. Br Med J 1990;300:64–622.
18 Liberato NL, Costa A, Barosi G: Erythropoietin: Biological aspects and clinical usefulness. Haematologica 1990;75:346–362.
19 Gregory CJ, Eaves AC: Human marrow cells capable of erythropoietic differentiation in vitro. Definition of three erythroid colony responses. Blood 1977;49:855–864.
20 Tepperman AD, Curtis JE, McColloch EA: Erythropoietic colonies in cultures of human marrow. Blood 1974;44:659–669.
21 Iscove NN, Gilbert LJ: Erythropoietin-independence of early erythropoiesis and a two-regulator model of a proliferative control in the hematopoietic system; in Murphy MJ Jr (ed): In vitro aspects of erythropoiesis. New York, Springer, 1978, pp 3–8.
22 Sieff CA, Emerson SG, Mufson A, Gesner TG, Nathan DG: Dependence of highly enriched human bone marrow progenitors on hemopoietic growth factors and their response to recombinant erythropoietin. J Clin Invest 1987;77:74–81.
23 Spivak JL: The mechanism of action of erythropoietin. Int J Cell Cloning 1986;4:139–166.
24 Zanjani ED, Lutton JD, Hoffman R, Wasserman LR: Erythroid colony formation by polycythemia vera bone marrow in vitro. Dependence on erythropoietin. J Clin Invest 1977;59:841–848.
25 Sonoda Y, Yang YC, Wong GG: Analysis in serum-free culture of the targets of recombinant human hematopoietic growth factors: Interleukin 3 and granulocyte macrophage colony-stimulating factor are specific for early development stages. Proc Natl Acad Sci USA 1988;85:4360–4364.
26 Ganser A, Holzer D: In vitro and in vivo regulation of erythro-

poiesis; in Jelkmann W, Gross AJ (eds): Erythropoietin. Berlin, Springer, 1989, pp 165–175.
27 Dessypris EN, Graber SE, Krantz SB, Stone WJ: Effects of recombinant erythropoietin on the concentration and cycling status of human marrow hematopoietic progenitor cells in vivo. Blood 1988;72:2060–2062.
28 Geissler K, Stockenhuber F, Kabrna E, Hinterberger W, Balcke P, Lechner K: Recombinant human erythropoietin and hematopoietic progenitor cells in vivo. Blood 1989;73:2229.
29 Mayeux P, Billant C, Jacquot R: Murine erythroleukemia cells (Friend cells) possess high affinity binding sites for erythropoietin. Fed Eur Biochem Soc 1987;211:229–233.
30 Sawyer ST, Krantz SB, Goldwasser E: Binding and receptor-mediated endocytosis of erythropoietin in Friend virus-infected erythroid cells. J Biol Chem 1987;262:5554–5562.
31 Fukamachi H, Tojo A, Saito T: Internalization of radioiodinated erythropoietin and the ligand-induced modulation of its receptor in murine erythroleukemia cells. Int J Cell Cloning 1987;5:209–219.
32 Sawada K, Krantz SB, Sawyer ST: Quantitation of specific binding of erythropoietin to human erythroid colonyforming cells. J Cell Physiol 1988;137:337–345.
33 Sawyer ST, Krantz SB, Goldwasser E: Binding and receptor-mediated endocytosis of erythropoietin in Friend virus-infected erythroid cells. J Biol Chem 1987;262:5554–5562.
34 Shaw AB: Haemolysis in chronic renal failure. Br Med J 1967; ii:213–216.
35 Lindsay RM, Burton JA, King P, Davidson JF, Boddy K, Kennedy AC: The measurement of dialyser blood loss. Clin Nephrol 1973;1:24–28.
36 Bischel MD, Neiman RS, Berne TV, Telfer N, Lukes RJ, Barbour BH: Hypersplenism in the uremic hemodialyzed patient. Nephron 1972;9:146–161.
37 Short AIK, Winney RJ, Robson JS: Reversible microcytic hypochromic anaemia in dialysis patients due to aluminum intoxication. Proc Eur Dial Transplant Assoc 1980;17:226–233.
38 Eschbach JW, Adamson JW: Anaemia of end-stage renal disease (ESRD). Kidney Int 1985;28:1–5.
39 Eschbach JW, Egrie JC, Downing MR: Correction of the anemia of end-stage renal disease with recombinant human erythropoietin. N Engl J Med 1987;316:73–78.
40 Winearls EC, Oliver DO, Pippard MJ: Effect of human erythropoietin derived from recombinant DNA on the anaemia of patients maintained by chronic haemodialysis. Lancet 1986; ii:1175.
41 Bommer J, Alexiou C, Muller-Buhl U, Eifert J, Ritze E: Recombinant human erythropoietin therapy in haemodialysis patients: Dose determination and clinical experience. Nephrol Dial Transplant 1987;2:238–242.
42 Nielsen OJ, Thaysen JH: Response to erythropoietin in anemic haemodialysis patients. J Intern Med 1989;31:97–98.
43 Zins B, Drueke T, Zingraff J: Erythropoietin treatment in anaemic patients on haemodialysis. Lancet 1986;ii:1329.
44 Casati S, Passerini P, Campise MR: Benefits and risk of protracted treatment with human recombinant erythropoiesis in patients having haemodialysis. Br Med J 1987;295:1012–1020.
45 Stutz B, Rhyner K, Vogtli J, Binswanger U: Erfolgreiche Behandlung der Anämie bei Hämodialyse-Patienten mit rekombiniertem humanem Erythropoietin. Schweiz Med Wochenschr 1987;117:1397–1402.
46 Adamson JW: The promise of recombinant human erythropoietin. Semin Hematol 1989;26(suppl 2):5–8.
47 Ponticelli C, Casati S: Correction of anaemia with recombinant human erythropoietin. Nephron 1989;52:201–208.
48 Zehnder C, Blumberg A: Human recombinant erythropoietin treatment in transfusion dependent anemic patients on maintenance hemodialysis. Clin Nephrol 1989;31:35–39.
49 Rosenlof K, Gronhagen-Riska C, Sovijaervi A: Beneficial effects of erythropoietin on haematological parameters, aerobic capacity, and body fluid composition in patients on hemodialysis. J Intern Med 1989;226:311–317.
50 Mayer G, Thum J, Cada EM, Stummvoll HK, Graf H: Working capacity is increased following recombinant human erythropoietin treatment. Kidney Int 1988;34:525–528.
51 Schaefer RM, Kokot E, Wernze H, Geiger H, Heidlend A: Improved sexual function in hemodialysis patients on recombinant erythropoietin: A possible role for prolactin. Clin Nephrol 1989;31:1–5.
52 Low I, Grutzmacher P, Bergmann M, Schoeppe W: Echocardiographic findings in patients on maintenance hemodialysis substituted with recombinant human erythropoietin. Clin Nephrol 1989;31:26–30.
53 Eschbach JW, Egrie JC, Downing MR, Browne JK, Adamson JW: Correction of the anaemia of end-stage renal disease with recombinant human erythropoietin. Results of a combined phase I and II clinical trial. N Engl J Med 1987;316:73–78.
54 Cotes P, Pippard MJ, Reid CDL, Winearls CG, Oliver DO, Royston JP: Characterization of the anaemia of chronic renal failure and the mode of its correction by a preparation of human erythropoietin (r-HuEPO). An investigation of the pharmacokinetics of intravenous erythropoietin and its effects on erythrokinetics. Q J Med 1989;70:113–137.
55 Dessypris EN, Graber SE, Krantz SB: Effects of recombinant erythropoietin on the concentration and cycling status of human marrow hematopoietic progenitor cells in vivo. Blood 1988;72:2060–2062.
56 Stone WJ, Graber SE, Krantz SB: Treatment of the anemia of predialysis patients with recombinant human erythropoietin: A randomized, placebo-controlled trial. Am J Med Sci 1988; 296:171.
57 Eschbach JW: Recombinant human erythropoietin in anemia patients with end-stage renal disease. Results of a phase III multicenter clinical trial. Ann Intern Med 1989;111:992–1000.
58 Raine AEG: Hypertension, blood viscosity, and cardiovascular morbidity in renal failure: Implications of erythropoietin therapy. Lancet 1988;i:97–99.
59 Bund SJ, Heagerty A, Edmunds M, Walls J: Erythropoietin does not induce vasoconstriction directly in human subcutaneous resistance arterioles. Nephron 1989;53:173.
60 Winearls CG, Oliver DO, Pippard MJ, Reid C, Downing MR, Cotes PM: Effect of human erythropoietin derived from recombinant DNA on the anaemia of patients maintained by chronic haemodialysis. Lancet 1986;ii:1175–1178.
61 Canadian Erythropoietin Study Group. Associated between recombinant human erythropoietin and quality of life and exercise capacity of patients receiving haemodialysis. Br Med J 1990;300:573–578.
62 Eschbach JW, Kelly MR, Haley NR, Abels RI, Adamson JW: Treatment of the anemia of progressive renal failure with re-

combinant human erythropoietin. N Engl J Med 1989;321:158–163.
63 Lim VS, DeGowin RL, Zavala D: Recombinant human erythropoietin treatment in pre-dialysis patients. A double-blind placebo-controlled trial. Ann Intern Med 1989;110:108–114.
64 Kleinman S, Schweitzer U, Perdue ST, Bleifer H, Abels RI: The use of recombinant human erythropoietin in the correction of anemia in predialysis patients and its effect on renal function: A double-blind, placebo-controlled trial. Am J Kidney Dis 1989;14:486–495.
65 Bommer J, Ritz E, Weinreich T, Bommer G, Ziegler T: Subcutaneous erythropoietin. Lancet 1988;ii:406.
66 Macdougall IC, Roberts DE, Neubert P, Dharmasena AD, Coles GA, Williams JD: Pharmacokinetics of recombinant human erythropoietin in patients on continuous ambulatory peritoneal dialysis. Lancet 1989;i:425–427.
67 Stevens JM, Strong CA, Oliver DO, Winearls CG, Cotes PM: Subcutaneous erythropoietin and peritoneal dialysis. Lancet 1989;i:1388–1389.
68 Macdougall IC, Roberts DE, Neubert P, Dharmasena AD, Coles GA, Williams JD: Pharmacokinetics of recombinant human erythropoietin in patients on continuous ambulatory peritoneal dialysis. Lancet 1989;i:425–427.
69 Kickler TS, Spivak JL: Effect of repeated whole blood donations on serum immunoreactive erythropoietin levels in autologous donors. JAMA 1988;260:65–67.
70 Goodnough LT, Brittenham GM: Limitation of the erythropoietin response to serial phlebotomy: Implications for autologous blood donor programs. J Lab Clin Med 1990;115:28–35.
71 Goodnough LT, Rudnick S, Price TH: Increased preoperative collection of autologous blood with recombinant human erythropoietin therapy. N Engl J Med 1989;321:1163–1168.
72 Maeda H, Hitomi Y, Hirata R: Erythropoietin and autologous blood donation. Lancet 1989;ii:284.
73 Baer AN, Dessypris EM, Goldwasser E: Blunted erythropoietin response to anemia in rheumatoid arthritis. Br J Haematol 1987;66:559–564.
74 Cartwright GE: The anemia of chronic disorders. Semin Hematol 1966;3:351.
75 Schooley JC, Kullgren B, Allison AC: Inhibition by interleukin-1 of the action of erythropoietin on erythroid precursor and its possible role in the pathogenesis of hypoplastic anemias. Br J Haematol 1987;67:11–17.
76 Stastny P, Rosenthal M, Andreis M: Lymphokines in the rheumatoid joint. Arthritis Rheum 1975;18:237.
77 Ton P, Shore A, Leary P: Interleukin abnormalities in recently active rheumatoid arthritis. J Rheumatol 1984;11:593.
78 Means RT, Olson NJ, Krantz SB: Treatment of the anemia of rheumatoid arthritis with recombinant human erythropoietin: Clinical and in vitro results. Arthritis Rheum 1989;32:638.
79 Takashina N, Kondo M, Kashiwazaki S: Suppressed serum erythropoietin response to anemia and the efficacy of recombinant erythropoietin in the anemía of rheumatoid arthritis. J Rheumatol 1990;17:885–887.
80 Zucker S, Friedman S, Lysik RR: Bone marrow erythropoiesis in the anemia of infection, inflammation and malignancy. J Clin Invest 1974;53:1132–1138.
81 Backwill F, Osborne R, Burke F: Evidence of tumor necrosis factor production in cancer. Lancet 1987;ii:1229.
82 Roodman GD, Bird A, Hutzler D: Tumor necrosis factor-alpha and hematopoietic progenitors. Effects of tumor necrosis factor on the growth of erythroid progenitors CFU-E and BFU-E and the hematopoietic cell lines K562, HL60, and HEL cells. Exp Hematol 1987;15:928–935.
83 Blick M, Sherwin SA, Rosenblum M: Phase I study of recombinant tumor necrosis factor in cancer patients. Cancer Res 1987;47:2986–2989.
84 Miller B, Jones J, Piantadosi S, Abeloff D, Spivak L: Decreased erythropoietin response in patients with the anemia of cancer. N Engl J Med 1990;322:1688–1692.
85 Oster W, Herrmann F, Gamm H, Zeile G, Lindemann A, Muller G, Brune T, Kraemer HP, Mertelsmann R: Erythropoietin for the treatment of anaemia of malignancy associated with neoplastic bone marrow infiltration. J Clin Oncol 1990;8:956–962.
86 Ludwig H, Fritz E, Kotzmann H, Hocker P, Gisskinder H, Barnas U: Erythropoietin treatment of anaemia associated with multiple myeloma. N Engl J Med 1990;322:1693–1699.
87 Oster W, Herrmann F, Cicco A, Mertelsmann R: Erythropoietin prevents chemotherapy induced anemia. Blut 1990;60: 88–92.
88 Aoki I, Higashi K, Homori M, Chikazawa H, Ishikawa K: Responsiveness of bone marrow erythropoietic stem cells to recombinant human erythropoietin in vitro in aplastic anemia and myelodisplastic syndromes. Am J Hematol 1989;35:6–12.
89 Baines P, Bowen D, Jacobs A: Clonal growth of haematopoietic progenitor cells from myelodisplastic marrow in response to recombinant haemopoietins. Leuk Res 1990;14:247–253.
90 Isnard F, Baillou CL, Ghaffari S: Stimulation of erythropoiesis in patients with refractory anaemias by recombinant human erythropoietin. Blood 1989;74(suppl)327a.
91 Hirishima K, Bessho M, Susaki K, Nagashima M: Improvement of anemia by intravenous injection of recombinant erythropoietin in patients with myelodysplastic syndrome and aplastic anemia. Exp Haematol 1989;17:657.
92 Oster W, Herrman F, Mertelsmann R: Erythropoietin for the treatment of patients with anemia of malignancy; in Mertelsmann R, Herrmann F (eds): Hematopoietic Growth Factors in Clinical Applications. New York, Dekker, 1990, pp 141–148.
93 Fischl M: Recombinant human erythropoietin for patients with AIDS treated with Zidovudine. N Engl J Med 1990;322: 1488–1493.

Prof. P. Foa
Istituto di Scienze Mediche
Padiglione Granelli
Via F. Sforza 35
I–20122 Milano (Italy)

Current Studies in Hematology and Blood Transfusion
(ISSN 0258–0330), **No. 57**
Series Editors: A. Hässig, P. Lundsgaard-Hansen, Bern

Editor: U.E. Nydegger

Therapeutic Hemapheresis in the 1990s

While the major indications for standard plasmapheresis and cytoreduction are now well defined, therapeutic hemapheresis is currently moving through an important period of transition. Looking to the future, this volume focuses on recent innovations in technology and technique as well as new clinical applications. Invited international experts analyze the risks and benefits of plasma exchange (PE), summarize the state of the art of available removal systems, and evaluate PE as a mode of therapy in a variety of disorders. Interesting features of the book include the use of novel apheresis harness and equipment, experiences with immunoadsorption and low-density lipoprotein apheresis, and the application of PE in HIV-related syndromes. Supplemented by clear figures and tables, this text contains useful information not only for clinicians with an interest in internal medicine, hematology and immunology but also for operators and harness producers.

Contents

Therapeutic Apheresis in Perspective
Klein, H.G.: Apheresis in Transition

Plasmapheresis
Isbister, J.P.: The Risk/Benefit Equation for Therapeutic Plasma Exchange. Analysis of the Rationale for and the Safety Aspects of Therapeutic Plasma Exchange · *Nydegger, U.E., et al.:* Synergy between Plasma Exchange and Intravenous Immunoglobulin · *Sawada, K., et al.:* Available Removal Systems: State of the Art · *Corvetta, A., et al.:* Plasma Exchange in Thrombotic Thrombocytopenic Purpura · *Carol, W., et al.:* Plasma Exchange in Idiopathic Thrombocytopenic Purpura · *Mason, P.D.; Pusey, C.D.:* Plasma Exchange in Nephrological Diseases · *Uldry, P.A.; Steck, A.J.:* Plasma Exchange in Neurology · *Kiprov, D.D., et al.:* Therapeutic Apheresis in HIV-Related Syndromes · *Matsuo, H., et al.:* Plasmapheresis to Treat Human T Lymphotropic Virus Type I Associated Myelopathy · *Riesen, W.F.:* Experience with Low-Density Lipoprotein Apheresis by Polyclonal and Monoclonal Anti-Apolipoprotein B Antibodies and by Dextran Sulfate Cellulose · *Guillevin, L., et al.:* Viscosity as the Symptom Leading to Plasma Exchange · *Borberg, H., et al.:* The Current Status of Low-Density Lipoprotein Apheresis

Therapeutic Cytapheresis
Hamblin, T.J.: Ex vivo Activation and Retransfusion of White Blood Cells. The Immunotherapy of Cancer · *Beris, P.; Dornier, C.:* Prevention and Circumvention of Refractoriness to Platelet Transfusions

Fields of Interest
Hematology; Internal Medicine; Immunology; Infectious Diseases, Neurology

Current Studies in Hematology and Blood Transfusion, No. 57
Therapeutic Hemapheresis in the 1990s
Editor: Nydegger, U.E. (Bern)
X + 282 p., 51 fig., 48 tab., hard cover, 1990
SFr. 267.– / DM 320.– / £ 116.10 / US$ 213.75
US $ price for USA, £ price for UK only (subject to change)
ISBN 3–8055–5166–5

KARGER

KI 90586

Monographs in Virology (ISSN 0077–0965), **Vol. 18**
Series Editor: J.L. Melnick, Houston, Tex.

Human Immunodeficiency Virus: Innovative Techniques for Isolation and Identification

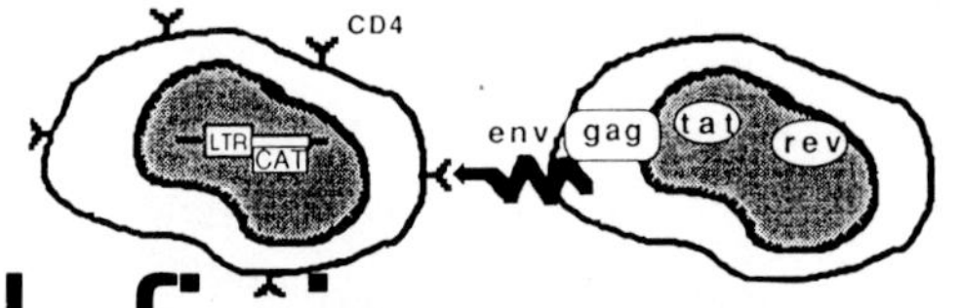

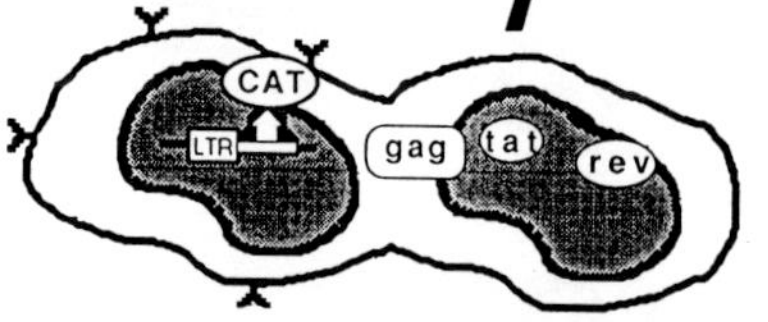

Editors:
N.C. Khan
J.L. Melnick

The humanimmunodeficiency virus (HIV) is the causative agent of acquired immunodeficiency syndrome (AIDS). Early detection of individuals infected with HIV enables the implementation of more effective measures to control and prevent the disease. This volume is concerned with recently developed techniques for the isolation and identification of HIV and for the monitoring of AIDS patients. Following an overview of HIV infection, leading investigators describe in detail innovative techniques for isolating the virus, for detecting viral nucleic acid and antigens, and for measuring a variety of antibodies associated with HIV.

Offering up-to-the-minute information plus a list of key references to the literature, this book provides virologists, immunologists, pathologists and clinical researchers with easy access to the most advanced techniques and views in this fast moving area of investigation.

Contents

Melnick, J.L.; Butel, J.S. (Houston, Tex.): An Overview of HIV Infection

Khan, N.C. (Rockville, Md.): Isolation of Human Immunodeficiency Virus from Infected Tissue Fluids, Tissues, and Cells

Keller, G .H.; Manak, M.M. (Rockville, Md.): Detection of HIV-1 Nucleic Acid in Clinical Samples Using Target DNA Amplification and Nonisotopic Probes

Krämer, A. (Bethesda, Md./Innsbruck) et al.: Levels of CD4+ Lymphocytes, Neopterin, and Beta-2-Microglobulin Are Early Predictors of Acquired Immunodeficiency Syndrome

Naylor, P.H. (Washington, D.C.) et al.: Diagnostic Assays for Human Immunodeficiency Virus Infection and for Clinical Progression by Use of Synthetic p17 Peptide Epitopes

Felber, B.K. (Frederick, Md.) et al.: Bioassays for the Detection of HIV-1 and Practical Applications

Devare, S.G. (Abbott Park, Ill.) et al.: Diagnosis and Monitoring of HIV-1 and HIV-2 Infection

Dimitrov, D.H.; Melnick, J.L.; Hollinger, F.B. (Houston, Tex.): Isolation of HIV-1 and Titration of Infected Peripheral Blood Mononuclear Cells by Microculture

Fields of Interest
Infectious Diseases; Immunology; Microbiology; Biochemistry, Epidemiology, Molecular Biology, Oncology, Virology

Monographs in Virology, Vol. 18
Human Immunodeficiency Virus: Innovative Techniques for Isolation and Identification
Editors: Khan, N.C. (Rockville, Md.); Melnick, J.L. (Houston, Tex.)
X + 130 p., 31 fig., 14 tab., hard cover, 1990
SFr. 134.– / DM 160.– / £ 58.30 / US$ 107.25
US$ price for USA, £ price for UK only (subject to change)
ISBN 3-8055-5182-7

KARGER

KI 90588